MAX YOUR MIND

Bless Your Beautiful
Brains!

Sandra Stanton

"The brain is the most intricate and delicate muscle of human anatomy—and perhaps the most precious of our God-given gifts. In *Max Your Mind*, Sandra Stanton brings it front and center and reveals it to be an important hinge for the door of our lives. Highlighting its connection with our bodies, spirits, and relationships, she offers practical advice and helpful exercises to keep it in tiptop shape. Learning from *Max Your Mind* will keep this important hinge from squeaking and rusting out."

—**Albert Haase**, OFM
Author of *Catching Fire, Becoming Flame: A Guide for Spiritual Transformation*

"Max Your Mind was a great encouragement to me. This book will provide information and inspiration for all who want to remain open to 'God's surprises.'"

—**Eric Alfrey**
Children's Minister, First Baptist Church, Columbia, SC
Former Director of Kunming International Academy, Kunming, China

"In *Max Your Mind*, author Sandra Stanton's enthusiasm for the subject of brain health really shines through. The information is accessible and very easy to grasp—just the perfect amount to be useful but not to overwhelm. The Reflections and Applications at the end of each chapter help make the material personally relevant to readers, helping them remember what they have learned and how to use it in everyday life."

—**Ann Brand**, Ph.D.
Instructor at University of Wisconsin–Stout

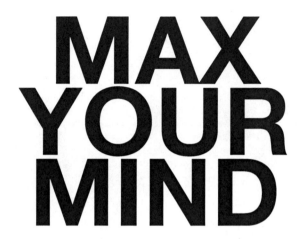

MAX YOUR MIND

The Owner's Guide for a Strong Brain

SANDRA SUNQUIST STANTON

New York

MAX YOUR MIND

The Owner's Guide for a Strong Brain

Published in New York, New York, by Morgan James Publishing. Morgan James and The Entrepreneurial Publisher are trademarks of Morgan James, LLC.
www.MorganJamesPublishing.com

The Morgan James Speakers Group can bring authors to your live event. For more information or to book an event visit The Morgan James Speakers Group at www.TheMorganJamesSpeakersGroup.com.

The information contained in this guide is not intended nor implied to be a substitute for professional medical advice; it is provided for educational purposes only. Nothing contained in this guide is intended to be used for medical diagnosis or treatment. Connections of the Heart doesn't endorse any product or company listed in this book, and expressly disclaims liability for any product, manufacturer, distributor, service, or service provider mentioned.

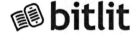

A **free** eBook edition is available
with the purchase of this print book.

CLEARLY PRINT YOUR NAME ABOVE IN UPPER CASE

Instructions to claim your free eBook edition:
1. Download the BitLit app for Android or iOS
2. Write your name in **UPPER CASE** on the line
3. Use the BitLit app to submit a photo
4. Download your eBook to any device

ISBN 978-1-63047-551-2 paperback
ISBN 978-1-63047-552-9 eBook
Library of Congress Control Number:
2015900216

Cover Design by:
Rachel Lopez
www.r2cdesign.com

Interior Design by:
Bonnie Bushman
bonnie@caboodlegraphics.com

In an effort to support local communities and raise awareness and funds, Morgan James Publishing donates a percentage of all book sales for the life of each book to Habitat for Humanity Peninsula and Greater Williamsburg.

Get involved today, visit
www.MorganJamesBuilds.com

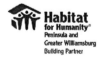

Habitat
for Humanity®
Peninsula and
Greater Williamsburg
Building Partner

*To God our Father, the Source of my inspiration
and Creator of our amazing brains and bodies.
And to Bob, my husband of 48 years, who has
honored my dream and made it his own.*

CONTENTS

Introduction

GOOD NEWS FOR
THE MATURING BRAIN!

Do any of these experiences sound familiar?

Why did I come into this room?
I spend way more time looking for things than I used to.
Her name is right on the tip of my tongue, but I can't pull it from my memory!

If so, you are not alone! Once we reach a certain age, "senior moments" seem to crop up more and more. The good news is that our understanding of *why* they crop up is also increasing more every day. Decades ago, scientists believed the brain peaked at age nineteen. More recently, they discovered that our brains are under construction until age twenty-five or later, when the brain cells in our prefrontal cortex (PFC)—that part of the brain behind the forehead—become fully protected by myelin. Our PFC is where self-control, planning, and "executive function" reside.

As we all know, our brains do indeed "fade" as we grow older, specifically in the areas of working memory, processing speed, word retrieval, remembering where we learned something, and detail discrimination. Multitasking makes us forget what we did or said. We have only one "main monitor," so as we age, we must choose our focus carefully.

But did you know that certain mental abilities actually get *better* with age? It's true! For example, our vocabulary and language skills grow with use. We're better able to pay attention to things that interest us. Our reasoning and ability to manage our emotions improve with use and maturity. Our dedication and willpower get stronger over time. Years of experience and broader perspective help us make better decisions, allowing both creativity and wisdom to blossom.[1] We can celebrate and appreciate these God-given abilities and use them to create more satisfying lives.

Hold on for the best part—in addition to the natural "fade" and "boost" the brain experiences with age, it continues to grow, change, and reorganize itself through our entire lives *based on our choices*: food, mental and physical exercise, musical training and expression, time and activities with friends, learning a new language, meditation, and even some video games have been proven to help use and strengthen the new brain cells our brain is constantly developing. New insights about *neuroplasticity*—our changing or "plastic" brain—have revised earlier research that told us we were "stuck" with the brain we had as young people. The brain is a "use it or lose it" organ, so with a little work, it can stay sharper than we may have thought.

I'd like to offer you some hope and encouragement to replace the disappointment and frustration you may experience when you forget things from time to time. In *Max Your Mind*, you'll learn to combat the natural "fade" in your brain that occurs over time and to "boost" the benefits. Think of it as an owner's manual for the fully myelinated brain, written particularly to help baby boomers, retirees, and those transitioning into retirement make sense of frustrating "senior moments" and deal positively with them.

My Lifelong Search for Answers

As a board-certified coach and speaker, people often ask me, "How did you get started with all this brain stuff?" I can trace my interest in the brain all the way back to age thirteen, when our family moved from Morris, Minnesota, to Cumberland, Wisconsin, in the middle of the school year. As a brand-new teenager in a brand-new town, I longed for the relationships and experiences I left behind, but was amazed at how I was able to carry complete images, experiences, and even close friendships with me—right in my own head! Replaying my multidimensional memories from Morris comforted me as I met and made new friends in the smaller but very friendly town of Cumberland.

The comfort of my vivid memories got me thinking: *How could my entire life be tucked away into my head? How could all the things my friends said and did—our routines, favorite songs, and private jokes—be saved in the small space between my ears? How was it possible for me to bring events back as though they were happening right now? How was I able to connect new experiences to the ones I left behind—only in my own mind?*

Our teacher Mrs. Gannon assigned a term paper that gave me the perfect chance to get my answers from my friend and librarian Katherine Robinson. Together we dug through the Cumberland Public Library's available encyclopedias and medical reference books, which had very little useful information. There wasn't much to begin with, and we felt as if we needed a translator to make sense of the material we did find.

That frustration led me on a lifelong search for answers about how the brain works. I've been blessed with both professional and volunteer training and experience during my journey. As an English teacher and school counselor, I was able to help students and families understand themselves and their experiences to become better prepared to make choices that fit their interests, skills, and preferences.

When our three daughters were born, I took ten years away from counseling to be with them during those developmentally critical first years. Our Catholic church in the 1970s had no programming for preschool children, so some other moms and I worked with the priests and sisters to set up a program for four- and five-year-olds. Social and spiritual growth during those early childhood years is so important to jumpstart their relationship skills.

A return to school counseling after my children were in school gave me an excellent arena to learn about the brain in order to help children, teachers, and families. I loved setting up programming for a positive school climate, which helped everyone associated with the school. As a member and eventually president of the Wisconsin School Counselor Association, I participated in ongoing training, networking across the country, and research and speaking opportunities, leading me to more answers about how the brain works.

After my retirement, Kunming International Academy, a 4K–12 school for the international community in China, asked me to help them set up a student records system. What a delight to be with children and families from twenty nations. Kids are the same everywhere! More on that adventure later.

In 2006, I set up my business, Connections of the Heart, LLC, and coined the term "brain coaching" to describe what has been my true work all along. I knew that the general public could benefit from the mountains of neuroscientific research, but most of it was written in terms only other neuroscientists used in their daily lives. Working with elementary school children and their families gave me opportunities to explain emerging information so it could be clear and useful to manage our lives and health, hence the name Connections of the Heart. It turns out our lives are most fulfilling and satisfying when our heart and brain work together, in "coherence."

Now I have the privilege of sharing my practical knowledge about the brain in classes and workshops for prenatal parents, infants, families, and retirees.

In individual brain coaching sessions, I support clients in transition as they work toward their chosen new "normal." We use tools to identify their preferred style for taking in new information and making decisions, and we do an energy audit to find out how they can best revitalize themselves. They identify goals and generate plans to reach them and consider options and obstacles. Working with motivated adults is my all-time favorite application of brain coaching. Cheering them on and watching them create fulfilling lives is an amazing blessing.

Connections of the Heart has taken me to eight states and Canada, as well as to local and regional seminars. My retired friends chide me for "flunking retirement." But sharing the answers to my lifelong questions is what truly lights up *my* brain (more on this in chapter 1).

My head is packed with so much information that it sometimes hurts! This project began fifteen years ago when I felt a nudge from God to put my studies into a book for others' benefit. Maya Angelou said it best: "There is no greater agony than bearing an untold story inside you." I'm relieved to get this story on paper so my work can help other adults. After morphing several times, this form is apparently the one God intended and has blessed. I am enormously thankful!

How to Max Your Mind

Max Your Mind will give you a basic overview of our brain's role in our lives based on the work of many researchers and scientists. Here I offer their findings in a conversational style, sprinkled with personal stories, to make the concepts as practical and as understandable as possible. Know that I am neither a neuroscientist nor lab researcher, merely someone with many questions about the brain and a lifelong hunger for the answers, which I am delighted to share with you.

Of course, scientists continue their quest to understand our amazing brains. God's design remains a challenge. The comprehensive explanation we're looking for is still a long way off, but new technology moves us closer every day. Also, more people than ever are fascinated with the connections between our mind, body, and spirit. As you will see, this book covers those topics as well.

Before we begin our journey together, the first thing to note is that the brain is not the same as the mind. I like Bob Goff's explanation from his book *Love Does:* "Psychologists are now theorizing about the separation of the brain and the mind. The brain is the stuff inside your skull. But the mind, they say, works a lot more like the Internet, a map of information collected from all our experiences and interactions with other people."[2]

Dr. Daniel Siegel has a more scientific explanation: "The mind is an embodied and relational process that regulates the flow of energy and information within the brain and between brains . . . extending throughout the entire body and also from the communication patterns that occur within relationships."[3]

So for the purposes of this book, the *brain* is the organ inside your skull, including not only its 100 billion brain cells and the trillions of connections between them, but all the axons that extend to the tips of your toes. The *mind* includes everything we take in through our senses, including our interactions with each other, with nature, and with the spiritual realm—however we define it.

Max Your Mind is divided into four main parts: Brain, Body, Spirit, and Relationships—which, taken together, comprise the experience of our mind. Each chapter closes with Reflections and Applications to help you apply a chapter's information in your own life. And each part includes a summary section to help you both "bless the boost" and "fight the fade" in your brain, body, spirit, and relationships. "Bless the Boost" will encourage you to make the most of those mental skills that actually improve with age, while "Fight the Fade" will give you specific tips to deal with the declining abilities you already know about.

Part Five will help you take action on what you've learned, with checklists and resources for folks who want to dig deeper about topics such as dementia or Alzheimer's, suggestions for further reading, and a repeat of all the Reflections and Applications from each chapter, in case you'd like to return to them later.

You can read the book cover to cover, or if you're looking for a quick read, you can use each section and/or chapter as a stand-alone reference. Please let me know how that works for you!

Remember, my research is mostly secondhand, studying the work of others and putting together personal observations and practical tips developed throughout my lifetime. My goal is to pass along clear, actionable information to people who want to understand and make the most of their own brains as they grow older and wiser. As we travel together on this quest to *Max Your Mind*, I would love to hear from you. Please feel free to e-mail me at sandra@sandrastantonauthor.com with your reactions, comments, and questions as you read this book.

I am immensely grateful that you have chosen to join me on this journey!

---

1   Aaron P. Nelson with Susan Gilbert, *The Harvard Medical School Guide to Achieving Optimal Memory* (McGraw-Hill, 2005), 51–52.

2   Bob Goff, *Love Does: Discover a Secretly Incredible Life in an Ordinary World* (Thomas Nelson, 2012), 118.

3   Daniel J. Siegel, *The Developing Mind: How Relationships and the Brain Interact to Shape Who We Are*, 2nd ed. (The Guilford Press, 2012), 3.

Part I
THE BRAIN

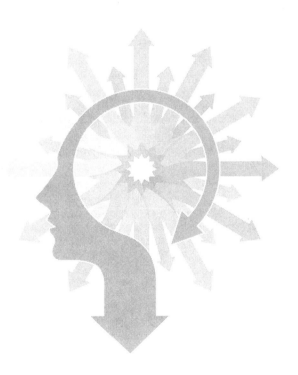

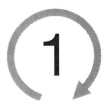

WHAT LIGHTS
UP YOUR BRAIN?

*What's your next step? . . . I bet it involves choosing something that
already lights you up. Something you already think is beautiful or lasting
and meaningful. Pick something that you aren't just able to do; pick
something that you feel that you were made to do and then do lots of that.*
—Bob Goff [1]

The mind is not a vessel to be filled, but a fire to be kindled.
—Plutarch

Your brain is a custom-designed gift, created by God, which allows you to learn and save information from your senses. With this data it goes to work developing your unique package of gifts and experiences. Your brain is not like anyone else's.

During our careers, to-do lists and expectations may have been imposed by "business interests," and retirement brings welcome new choices! It's time to find out what you were made to do! In this chapter, we will look at the ways some people have found fulfillment and have improved others' lives by recognizing what lights up their brain.

How Does My Brain Light Up?

Lighting up my brain? How is that possible? Since science has given us technology to look inside our brains, we can actually see what happens when we are excited about something we're doing. When we love what we're doing, our brains "light up." Researchers can now insert radioactive dye that migrates to the active parts of the brain during a given activity. They then conduct brain scans, using *functional magnetic resonance indicators* (fMRIs), to show increased blood flow in the areas we are using at that time. Those active areas appear to "light up" on scan results. Nope, our brains aren't really glowing—good thing!

God had a purpose in mind when he created us. When we stay tuned into him, he provides everything we need to accomplish that purpose. We could say that we were each "made to do" something special. When we discover and develop that God-given talent, we can feel the excitement that goes with fulfilling his purpose for our lives.

Creative Journeys

Discovering what you truly love to do may begin with looking at choices made by others in our lives. I've been inspired by the creativity of friends and relatives and the joy it brings into their lives. My friend Sue loves photography and painting with watercolors. She gave me one of her framed soft pastel paintings, which "happened" to perfectly match the colors of our bathroom. Another friend, Mary Jo, makes beautiful jewelry and knitted gifts. Her husband, Tom, retired Navy, discovered watercolor painting while we cruised together on the Seine River through France; his painting prowess continues to grow, and he loves it.

My brother-in-law Jerry says being "downsized" from his corporate job freed him up to do his own thing, which he calls "Interpretations in Hardwood." Jerry creates abstract eagles, wolves, and owls from hardwoods—bird's-eye maple, cherry, black walnut, ash, mahogany, western cedar, and others. A Harley-Davidson devotee, he and his wife Jill love open-air rides on their Harley-Davidson motorcycles, and their son has one, too. When Jerry showed his work to the iconic motorcycle company's decision makers, they chose him to create Harley-Davidson's commemorative centennial bronze eagle wall sculpture. That piece has been reproduced and sold around the world. [2]

Working with fabric while enjoying the company of friends has brought peace to women in particular for centuries. Mickey's brain lights up with her many quilting projects, and she and her group of quilting friends enjoy time together on their annual retreats. Another friend, Anne, has a designated quilting space in her home where she can focus her attention and energy on sewing while her stress melts away.

Close friends and retired educators, Pam, Ellen, Jane, and Jessie, have been embroidering and sewing together since I've known them. At Indianhead Embroidery Guild meetings, they taught me Hardanger embroidery, and I experienced the joy of exploring a new aspect of my Norwegian heritage. Their intricate needlework graces their own homes and those of many people they love. I was delighted to learn the craft and create small Hardanger baptismal keepsakes for my grandchildren.

Spinning and knitting is another way to "play." Barb and her husband Randy have raised Suri alpacas since she retired from teaching. They chose alpacas because of their silken, cashmere-soft fleece, which is warmer than wool. Working with the sweet, gentle animals and their high-end fleece brings her peace, and the rhythmic motion of spinning the fleece into yarn soothes her body and mind.

I interviewed another spinner, retired audiology professor Nan Weiler, who lived at the time in Wisconsin's north woods. "Every human being has his or her own way of expressing creativity; we need only to find it," Nan said. "Mine is spinning and working with fibers, but each person's search is different . . . . Sometimes you admire a piece of art and would like to create something similar. Sometimes you just want to improve on something you got somewhere else. Playing is very important for us mentally and physically. In the woods, we find that we can play all day. All this work with fiber is very productive play, but healthful play just the same." [3]

Diann, a retired counselor, plays the flute, and creates beautifully crafted papers and books. Her current passion is designing and making pottery. Friends don't mind waiting for the specially designed items she creates. As gifts or personal possessions, they carry the joy and peace she feels while making them.

Other retirees find joy in mentoring individuals beginning their career journeys, helping with nonprofit causes, or, in my case, writing. One of my first and still-favorite resources is *The Artist's Way* by Julia Cameron. Following the exercises in her book, I write "morning pages" at the start of my day when my thoughts are fresh and free. Stream-of-consciousness, longhand writing for three pages is best, she says, without our inner editor. This is great exercise for my creative right brain.[4] Neuroscientists agree. Activating eye/hand coordination, fine motor muscles, and the brain's creative process simultaneously develops strong connections between each of these mind-based functions. Repeat, repeat, repeat, and they become a team.

Writing is something I need to do every day. When I don't take the time to download my thoughts onto the page, my mind gets sluggish and foggy. Not everyone would understand, but it feels good to spend time with those who do. My first nudge to study *The Artist's Way* and endless other writers' tips came from Western Wisconsin Christian Writers Guild where I found kindred spirits and the encouragement to keep trying.

Since 2006, the Society of Children's Book Writers and Illustrators and my critique group have helped me develop my picture-book writing skills to reach the younger crowd with brain coaching stories. Two of my favorite creative writers, Anne Lamott[5] and Ann Voskamp,[6] inspire me to dig deeper and let my heart come out to play or cry. Writing can be an exercise in self-discovery. I'm often surprised at what I see on the page.

We don't have to save the world. Discovering what lights up our own brains is enough to get us started down a path of discovery or rediscovery.

Lighting Up Your Brain Can Light Up Others' Lives

But sometimes creativity does lead to lighting up someone else's life. Bob Goff, lawyer, speaker, and author of *Love Does* inspires me and many others to "Love

God, Love People, Do Stuff," as he wrote in my copy of his book. As the keynote speaker for the Second Wind conference at Peace Lutheran Church in Eau Claire, Wisconsin, he spoke with delight of "leaking Jesus in whimsical ways" and enjoyed calling his work a series of "capers" for God.

He shared a bit of background that helped us understand his passion. Bob Goff, of Goff and Dewalt, a West Coast law firm, is the father of three. After the World Trade Center 9/11 crisis, he asked his children what they would do if they had five minutes with a world leader. His seven-year-old wanted to invite the world leader to a sleepover. His nine-year-old wanted to ask what the world leader's hopes were, and perhaps pass his or her dreams on to other leaders. His oldest daughter was into video, so she wanted to ask those who weren't able to come for a sleepover if the Goff children could visit them in their home country and videotape interviews asking about their hopes.

The children wrote and sent personal letters to leaders of every nation, inviting them to the Goff home for a sleepover. Most sent kind regrets. Thirty-two leaders came for sleepovers to visit the children. Bob and his wife, whom he calls "Sweet Maria," served as observers and hosts.

Bulgaria was the first of twenty-nine invitations the family received, inviting them to their home country for an interview. As promised, Bob took his children on a whirlwind trip to these twenty-nine regal homes, and the kids got the chance to ask their questions.

During their tour of nations, they discovered children being sold as commodities on the black market to slave camps in Mumbai, India. Bob and his children wanted to make a difference for children who were the same age as they were.

Similar travesties showed up in African nations, leading Bob and his family to focus their attention on Uganda, where the average age was 14 after the loss of many lives during a violent war in the northern part of the country. The country was experiencing an enormous backlog of court cases. Hundreds had been accused and had to wait two to three years in prison before they set foot in a Kampala, Uganda, courtroom.

In response to the incredible need, Bob and his colleagues created Restore International to defend and rescue the children. Lawyers and law students from

Pepperdine University and Seattle University took up Bob's charge. Together, they worked within the Ugandan legal system and freed seventy-two children, returning them to their parents. After several months, all charges had been dropped or otherwise resolved.

In 2007, they built the Restore Leadership Academy, a secondary school for the children in Gulu, Uganda, many of whom were former child soldiers, orphans, or victims of sex trafficking or extreme poverty. At first, they struggled to get students, opening the school with eighteen teachers and nine kids. On October 27, 2009, all 230 enrolled students attended the school's graduation of seventeen students.[7]

Their efforts were so appreciated that Uganda's Prime Minister, Apolo Nsibambi, ultimately named Bob the Honorary Consul for the Republic of Uganda to the United States. He travels to Uganda every one hundred days to try more cases and free the innocent.[8]

During his live presentation at Peace, Bob shared another true story of Ugandan witch doctors who had been mutilating young boys as sacrifices. Restore International has successfully rescued hundreds of boys, and the Goffs adopted one of them and arranged for his reconstructive surgery. This led to the creation of Bob's Witch Doctor School, which uses only the *Bible* and *Love Does* as curriculum.[9] In his "capers" following God's nudges to help others, Bob also lights up others' lives on a grand scale!

Of course, not everyone can expect to have this kind of impact. In an interview Bob did for *60 Minutes,* he said, "It just sounds like you're blowing sunshine at people, saying: 'You can do anything.' And it's . . . true, in a sense, but it just sounds unrealistic. What I think anybody can be is engaged. And so, we're all given this unique wiring harness—you have one, I have one, everybody has this unique wiring harness. And so then you think, how could you live into that?"[10]

Seeking and identifying our "unique wiring harness" may take time and energy, as well as an understanding that our everyday tasks are truly important. Retirees may find it easier to observe others' gifts than to zero in on their own. Many of us are caregivers for family members with health issues, and our responsibilities seem overwhelming. We try to help others when they need it, but we haven't given any thought to lighting up our own brains. It somehow seems selfish. Not so!

When we find and enthusiastically pursue our passion—even in daily chores—our energy, health, spirit, and relationships benefit. To echo Bob Goff, who uses a chess game analogy, "Take the smallest piece and move it one square toward Jesus."[11]

What if you haven't taken the time to develop your gift—and frankly, you're not very good at it? Is it too late? The answer is a definite no, thanks to the magic of *neuroplasticity*.

Neuroplasticity

What a relief to discover that my high school biology teacher was wrong! Of course, he taught us from current science that our brains peaked at age nineteen—which felt like the distant future to us at the time—and everything would go downhill from there. In his defense, he didn't have the benefit of the growing body of information we have today.

Our scientific understanding of our God-created human brain has come a long way. A *National Geographic* article, "Secrets of the Brain," helps us understand what's going on inside our heads. Ancient scientists first thought the brain was made up of "phlegm," then "vapors." Eventually, they discovered the electrical nature of the brain, with its 100,000 miles of nerve fibers connecting brain cells and other components.

In recent decades, researchers have been able to use fMRIs and *single photon emission computed tomography* (SPECT) scans to study the inside of the brain while it's working. Researchers now hope to create maps of the brain, which will eventually help doctors diagnose and treat cognitive diseases.[12] One of the concepts that has developed from this increased understanding is *neuroplasticity*.

Neuroplasticity is an odd term for most people. It has nothing to do with food storage or recycling efforts. It's actually one of the most hopeful concepts I've run across in a long time. Dr. Richard Davidson, University of Wisconsin-Madison researcher, defines neuroplasticity as the brain's "ability to change its structure and patterns of activity in significant ways not only in childhood, which is not very surprising, but also in adulthood and throughout life. That change can come about as a result of experiences we have as well as of purely internal mental activity—our thoughts." [13]

It means we're not stuck with our nineteen-year-old brains. Our brains are capable of producing new neurons and connections throughout our lifetimes. Any time we find a new way to connect our existing brain cells, we build new skills. With repetition and consistent effort, we can fulfill our dreams! A recent news item featured a woman who wrote a book at age ninety-nine and is planning a book tour when she's one hundred.

Bottom line—neuroplasticity gives our brains the opportunity to continue to create new cells and connections throughout our entire lifetime, as long as we give them what they need. Like the muscles in our bodies, our brains need to be stretched and challenged to stay sharp.

Neurobics

When we can't remember an actor's name or the person who referred us to a particular restaurant, it's easy to panic. "I'm losing my mind!" we think. "Maybe I've got Alzheimer's!" Actually, as we grow older, the connections that reach from one brain cell to another may simply be getting weaker from lack of exercise or from not being "switched on" as much. This phenomenon has more in common with physical exercise than we might expect. Just as we need to exercise many different muscle groups for optimal physical health (known as creating "muscle confusion"—the principle behind circuit training), we can keep our brain cells and dendrites in optimal by using them in new ways. Lawrence Katz calls this kind of brain exercise *Neurobics*. The similarity to "aerobics" is no accident.

Dr. Katz's book *Keep Your Brain Alive* gives us eighty-three simple ways to keep our brain cells communicating with each other and creating new connections. Writing with your non-dominant hand is just one example, but there are many more. According to Dr. Katz, Neurobic exercises have three criteria: [14]

1. Use one or more of your senses in an unusual way or combination. For example:
   - Get dressed or brush your teeth with your eyes closed.
   - Combine two or more senses in unexpected ways. Choose a scent to pair with a particular piece of music.
2. Trigger your full attention. For example:
   - Wear a wrist or knee brace to work for a day to wake up your kinesthetic sense.
   - Search for keys in a purse using only your senses of touch and hearing.
3. Switch up the way you accomplish a routine activity. For example:
   - Take a completely new route to work.
   - Shop at a farmers market or flea market.

Neurobics, then, refers to any brain exercise that can either wake up sluggish neurons or create brand new connections.

Another more challenging exercise is to focus on our body's senses in the present moment, which can help manage our negative emotions. Many of us get caught up in feelings about events and actions of the past or fear of what may be ahead. We may need a nudge to shift our focus from those feelings—which are not facts—so we can tune into what's actually happening in and around us. We'll talk more about that in chapter 4. For now, here are some personal stories to illustrate the process based on my own experiences.

Staying Open to God's Surprises

God gives us enough grace for today, but we can't stockpile it for tomorrow. We're told to keep our focus on the space we can see—like a flashlight on our path. Trying to outrun that light only leads to trouble. God is enough, and I thank him for that lesson. Our experiences of joy need to be new every day, just like the manna God gave to the Israelites in the desert.

God constantly reaches out to us with his gifts, but if we're stuck in past regrets or future worries, we will miss them. Spencer Johnson's classic,

The Precious Present, [15] reminds us that this moment is precious; that's why it's called the present. We can remember what it was like yesterday and anticipate tomorrow's excitement, but the brain only lights up *now*. We can't be truly alive clinging to yesterday or tomorrow. It's all about our senses and the messages they send to our brains.

As I practiced being present with my Hmong students as a school counselor at Longfellow Elementary School, their stories touched me deeply. These refugee families risked their lives, leaving family and friends to come to the United States and fulfill their dreams. They would tell me how they used plastic bags as rafts to cross the Mekong River. I became obsessed with these stories and longed to go to Thailand and dip my own hand in the river to honor their struggle.

In 2005, that dream came true for me. Suzan Nolan, my fellow state counselor, association president, and friend from South Dakota, invited me to join a group from her church traveling to Bangkok, Chiang Mai, Chiang Rai, and the Thai hill country. We visited the New Life Center in Chiang Mai, a boarding school for young hill country women who were at risk of human trafficking because they were unable to take the citizenship exam without knowing the classic Thai language. All legitimate employment required official citizenship papers. They learned the language and exquisite Thai needlework at the Center. [16]

I felt God nudging me to bring that story home, along with my own adventure of reaching the Mekong. Upon my return home, the New Life Center's director and I collaborated on an article describing the school for the *Eau Claire Leader-Telegram.* That article made its way to China and to Eric Alfrey, director of Kunming International Academy (KIA). He read the article, Googled me, and called to ask me to come to China to help them lay the groundwork for a student records system so graduates could meet application requirements to attend university programs around the world.

My husband and I asked many questions before accepting that assignment, but God's timing and provisions made it a reality in record time. We felt peace and trust rather than fear or worry, even though I would be traveling alone in a foreign environment. Staying in the moment and trusting God for the outcome made the experience both fulfilling and productive. It was the trip of a lifetime for me.

As mentioned earlier, KIA is a 4K–12 school serving the international community in Kunming, China, and is organized under the Oasis International Schools, a division of the Network of International Christian Schools, based in the United States. The Chinese government prohibits Chinese children from attending KIA. Students came from twenty countries and various school backgrounds, and they wanted post-secondary education from various universities around the world. The school needed a consistent system to prepare their students' academic transcripts for applications. Again, God took care of the details, and I spent the rest of their school year living with Jean Bannen in China and working with all 4K-12 classes at KIA. The staff achieved full accreditation a couple of years later.

God's love was palpable in the KIA school family. To me, the experience felt like riding a surfboard—absolutely no control, but clearly safe and guided step-by-step by my KIA friends and our amazing God. I will be forever grateful for that experience and hope my time there was helpful to them, serving his purposes.[17]

I lived in the present moment each day in China. Getting to school and back and daily tasks took my full attention. God provided everything I needed, and things I didn't know I wanted, through the dear people of KIA. Every day brought new experiences. I learned to stay open to God's surprises and trust him for everything. That lesson is still with me today, ten years later. I love being teachable and filled with gratitude—even for the challenges.

What about My Brain?

So where do we go with all this? What does it look like, specifically, in each of our lives?

With medical advances, our "second act" after retirement will probably be longer than that of our grandparents.[18] Coasting to the finish doesn't seem like a healthy option. Identifying activities that light up our brains will add richness to our remaining years on this earth. I often ask clients and audiences to list three things they already do that light up their lives. I'll share some of their examples as stepping stones for your search.

- Playing, listening, telling stories with grandchildren
- Fixing things—not practical, physical things, but taking on problems and resolving them
- Gardening
- Rescuing and rehabilitating dogs
- Writing and telling joyful stories
- Writing to encourage Christ's followers
- Laughing
- Playing
- ~~Golf~~ Practicing patience [I can relate!]
- Sewing
- Sketching
- Helping my mother recover with play and laughter
- Finding humor
- Keeping a gratitude list
- Flower arranging
- Designing and developing landscape plans
- Reading
- Writing/blogging
- Helping/serving others
- Practicing hospitality
- Parenting children
- Spending time with friends
- Serving at community food banks
- Being outside
- Being with people
- Working in nursing
- Showing empathy
- Learning things I didn't know before
- Doing anything outdoors

- Playing or listening to music
- Playing guitar
- Cooking
- Nurturing relationships—listening, learning
- Building strong friendships and family ties
- Caregiving with quality time
- Taking classes with friends
- Enjoying good health
- Sharing God's grace
- Knowing God loves me
- Nurturing and encouraging
- Caring for people
- Running for charity
- Hunting
- Bookkeeping
- Dancing
- Making gifts
- Exercising
- Worshipping
- Spending time with horses
- Connecting a fourteen-year-old girl to her passion for horses as she deals with her life challenges

Their list intrigued me, with its variety and depth of involvement. It illustrates the many different paths God has for us when we trust him.

If you aren't sure what activities truly light up your brain, take advantage of the opportunities retirement offers! You may want to explore something completely different from your career skills. If you've always worked with data, try creating with your hands. Exercising the non-dominant side of your brain can be very satisfying, and it keeps your brain growing and healthy.

Getting back to Bob Goff's charge for us: "Just like God's Son arrived here, so did you. And after Jesus arrived, God whispered to all of humanity, 'It's your move.'" [19]

"Jesus doesn't invite us on a business trip. Instead, he says let's go after those things that inspire and challenge you and let's experience them together. You don't need a lot of details or luggage or equipment, just a willingness to go into a storm with a Father who's kicking footholds into the steep sides of our problems while we kick a couple in ourselves too. He guides us into those footholds with his strong hands while we're safely tethered to him by a bright red rope of grace, which holds us securely." [20]

Our brains have the amazing capability to bundle our feelings, relationships, environment, risks, opportunities, and memories to make us unique. They are way more complex than any computer, with amazing gifts we are just beginning to understand.

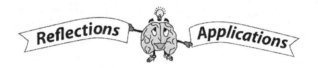

Reflection

Do you believe God created you with special gifts? They are blessings from God to bring satisfaction and joy to your life and the lives of others.

Application

1. List three things you were "made" to do.
2. As a Neurobics exercise, share a meal with family or friends with the radio, TV, cell phones, and all other electronic devices turned off. Focus your attention on your conversation and the taste and texture of the food.
3. Discuss any differences between the electronic-free meal and your usual dining experience.

---

1   Goff, *Love Does*, 216.
2   Sandra Sunquist Stanton, "Stanton Works: Downsized to a Harley-Davidson Upgrade," *Wisconsin West*, August 2003, 15–17.
3   Sandra Sunquist Stanton, "Spinning a Northwood's Peace," *Wisconsin West*, December 2001, 20–23.

4   Julia Cameron, *The Artist's Way: A Spiritual Path to Higher Creativity* (Tarcher/ Perigree, 1992), 10–18.

5   Anne Lamott, *Help, Thanks, Wow: The Three Essential Prayers* (Riverhead Books, 2012).

6   Ann Voskamp, *One Thousand Gifts: A Dare to Live Fully Right Where You Are* (Zondervan, 2010).

7   For more information about Restore Leadership Academy, see http:// restoreinternational.org/restoreleadershipacademy/.

8   Katie Conner, "Bob Goff *60 Minutes*," https://www.youtube.com/ watch?v=TDJHfRntv0M.

9   You can read more about Bob Goff's ministry at http://restoreinternational.org/ witchdoctorschool/.

10 Katie Conner, "Bob Goff *60 Minutes*," https://www.youtube.com/ watch?v=TDJHfRntv0M.

11 Bob Goff, Keynote Address at Second Wind Conference, Peace Lutheran Church, Eau Claire, Wisconsin, April 5, 2014.

12 Carl Zimmer, "Secrets of the Brain: New Technologies Are Shedding Light on Biology's Greatest Unsolved Mystery: How the Brain Really Works," *National Geographic*, February 2014, 28–57.

13 Richard Davidson and Sharon Begley, *The Emotional Life of Your Brain: How Its Unique Patterns Affect the Way You Think, Feel, and Live—and How You Can Change Them* (Hudson Street Press, 2012), 161.

14 Lawrence C. Katz and Manning Rubin, *Keep Your Brain Alive: 83 Neurobic Exercises to Help Prevent Memory Loss and Increase Mental Fitness* (Workman, 1999), 34.

15 Spencer Johnson, *The Precious Present* (Doubleday, 1984).

16 Sandra Sunquist Stanton, "Cultural Exchange: An Eau Claire Woman Visited a Thailand Center That Helps Young Women Adjust to Life Outside Their Tribal Villages but Retain Their Heritage," *Leader-Telegram*, March, 2005, D1.

17 Sandra Sunquist Stanton, "To China with Love: An Eau Claire Counselor Serves at a Christian School," *Leader-Telegram*, October 15, 2005, D1.

18 Jane Pauley, "Second Acts: Life Is Long. Yours May Be Overdue for an Overhaul," *Time*, June 30, 2014, 46.

19 Goff, *Love Does*, 217.

20 Ibid., 133.

BRAIN BASICS

*No computer can match the human brain
for its complexity and its potential for creative thought.*
—Michael S. Sweeney[1]

My passion for communication has always puzzled my friends and colleagues. Let me try to help you appreciate it. First, we get to store our entire world of experience within the three-pound mass of tissue between our ears. After we add our own spin to everything we keep, we translate these thoughts, memories, and images into words or pictures that could generate similar concepts in another's consciousness. Next, the listener or reader chooses what to take in and then make it her own. Our shared memories become the foundation for relationships that can last a lifetime. God put us together in amazing ways that we're just beginning to understand. What a trip!

In this chapter, we'll discover basic neuroscience principles, the specific parts of the brain, and how these parts work together. "Brain coaching" for me means helping people clearly understand how the brain works so they can make better everyday choices and decisions. The term "life coaching" has become widely understood, referring to individual coaching about life decisions. With individual brain coaching clients, we apply these concepts to help them identify and reach their chosen goals and issues, referring to relevant brain functioning to help them understand what's happening in their lives. When I present brain coaching workshops, articles, and books, I focus on issues relevant to a targeted group—adults, moms, parents, teens, seniors, educators, and others. Whether it's working with individuals or speaking to groups, the theme is basic neuroscience described in familiar terms.

The findings of neuroscientists are available in countless published journals, but this is not the typical reading material most of us would choose. I like to translate their work into usable tips for those of us struggling with the "fade" of aging.

Ever "lost" your keys? Ever tried to figure out why, so you can prevent it from happening again? To illustrate the need for clear communication, and why brain coaching can be so helpful, I'll share just a short part of an explanation in *Science Blog*. I believe you will see why not everyone can easily make the leap from research language to actionable tips.

In this example, neuroscientists begin to describe what actually happens in the brain: "Laboratory studies found that in fact the same populations of neurons in the dentate gyrus are active in different environments, and that the way the cells distinguished new surroundings was by changing the rate at which they sent electrical impulses. This discrepancy between theoretical predictions and laboratory findings has perplexed neuroscientists and obscured our understanding of memory formation and retrieval." [2]

We could go on, but I think you get the idea. To understand something we read, it must connect to something we already have stored in our memories. That blog I quoted above was written to explain brain processes to people who use neuroscience terms regularly, as a part of their work; brain coaching can help us translate the findings from a lengthy article and come up with practical suggestions, which might go something like this:

To have more success finding your keys when you need them, you can change some simple habits.

1. Try putting your keys in the same place every time. A basket or hook works great.
2. Say aloud where you are putting them. When you hang them up, talk to yourself, to activate both speech and hearing: "My keys are on the second hook from the left." This brings the action to your "main monitor" and away from autopilot, engaging the brain in the process. Involving as many senses as possible increases the likelihood of remembering later.
3. Visualize them hanging from the light switch below the hook.

This process works because you are making the "memory" multidimensional, with sensory "handles," so it's easier to grab that memory when we need it.

With that example of brain coaching, you at least have some suggestions of ways to make your way out the door more quickly—with less time searching for those darn keys. Whether these suggestions actually help us create new habits depends on your own motivation to make changes. Our choices and feelings can propel us forward or hold us back, as always.

Emotions also can sidetrack problem solving—and they're often a part of the problem. As a school counselor, I remember problem solving sometimes stalled when children had conflicts with each other or when family members had difficulty seeing the problem from the other person's perspective. When someone got stuck, I often shifted to using basic neuroscience to explain the situation. Working with objective information made blame and shame less likely to short-circuit solutions. Brain coaching—sharing a practical understanding of how the brain works and what it needs—helped us come up with solutions that all parties could more easily accept. The same principles that I used with schoolchildren apply to adults. Specifically:

- Fear shuts down our ability to think. We must find ways to calm the mind before we can expect to absorb new information or connect with what we have already learned.
- Mutual support and fun improve the likelihood of successful learning. The brain works best when it feels supported.
- Adding music uses both sides of the brain, giving memories depth and richness, making them easier to recall later.
- Breaks give the brain's synapses a chance to absorb information. It works like setting Jell-O® or cement. A short rest works to lock in the connections after we learn something new. Anyone missing those kindergarten naps?

The body also needs to move every ten to twenty minutes in order for the brain to learn best—at any age. I like the way another educator put it: "When the bum is numb, the brain is the same." Providing movement breaks makes learning easier in any situation.

Physical activity actually increases the formation of brain cells and connections. Get moving to max your brain. Teachers have told me that they plan an outdoor run or walk to boost their students' ability to think before tough tasks. Recess, anyone? It improves performance every time. Many teachers plan short bursts of movement into their students' day and are amazed at the positive differences in both performance and behavior. Brain Gym® is a collection of exercises used for decades to boost alertness and performance in classrooms.[3]

It works for me, too. My dog seems to know when I become bogged down during long writing sessions. She comes to nudge me, and we take a walk. The exercise break gives me fresh thoughts and ideas—and a happy dog! More about this in chapter 5.

Your Brain by the Numbers

Our brain is composed of 100 billion neurons. To visualize that number, a stack of 100 billion pieces of paper, laid on its side, would extend from San Francisco, all the way across the United States and the Atlantic Ocean, to London. One would think so many cells would be able to accomplish a great deal, but that can't happen without the connections to enable them to work together. Imagine trying to place a phone call to your sister in Minneapolis. Without refined connections, every phone in the city would ring—not just your sister's phone. How confusing that would be!

Connections form when two different cells become active at the same time. Scientists offer this explanation: "Cells that fire together—wire together." Linked in countless sequences based on our experiences, each cell can connect to thousands of others throughout our brain. Together, they create infinite possibilities.

The brain grows from bottom to top, back to front, and inside to outside. At birth, a baby has 50 trillion synapses, but by age three, that child has 1,000 trillion synapses, about twice as many as her pediatrician.[4] During the following years, the brain prunes the unused connections to make room for complex networks that it will need later.

Behind the forehead, we find the most sophisticated part of the brain. The *prefrontal cortex* (PFC) is what we use when we plan, set goals, exercise self-control, consider consequences, and put off doing or getting something we want. It's the location of our conscience and the seat of our higher thinking skills, or executive function.[5]

One of the most startling facts I've run across lately came from Dr. Caroline Leaf: as adults our brains process *400 billion bits of information every second* to keep our bodies functioning.[6] Remember that when you wonder where your headache came from. All this happens completely without our awareness in the amazing brain God created. It blows my mind!

Can you believe the ways our lives have changed through human brains working with technology? Some say computers have revolutionized our world, but our brains are even more complex—and science has still to complete mapping of the brain.

Brain versus Computer

Some people like to be able to hold, smell, and personalize a printed book. Others prefer the easy access of electronic storage. Early in computer development, some alluded to the computer as an electronic brain. They serve some of the same purposes, but the comparison falls apart along the way.

Unlike a computer, which saves huge numbers of individual facts or figures, the human brain records memories as complex packages with pieces all over the brain. They include pictures, words, colors, sounds, and especially emotions, which we are able to bring back on demand. Our feelings and experiences create changes in our memories each time we remember them.

Tim Berners-Lee, the creator of the World Wide Web, gives us a quick description of how memory works: "A piece of information is defined only by what it's related to. The structure is everything. Billions of neurons populate our brains, but what are neurons? Just cells . . . . The brain has no knowledge until connections exist between neurons. All we know, all that we are, comes from the way our neurons are connected."[7]

The Way It Works—at the Cellular Level

Our five senses gather information and send it to the brain cells designed to receive each particular type of input. *Dendrites* receive it first. Activated neurons then pass it along through the *axon*, where *neurotransmitters* either boost or slow the process to the next brain cell. Most of the work actually happens in the *synapses*—the space between brain cells. This system grows and multiplies, creating connections and networks that become stronger and more complex with repeated use.[8]

While the brain works together as a whole organ, it's easier to understand by looking at its levels, parts, and their functions. David J. Linden, PhD, a Johns Hopkins University neuroscientist and author of *The Compass of Pleasure,* compares the levels of the brain to an ice cream cone. The simpler, more primitive parts are placed at the bottom, and we build it adding more complex "scoops" one at a time. According to Linden, "lower parts like the cerebellum and hypothalamus, which handle survival-oriented behavior like sex drive and eating, haven't evolved as much, so what the lizard has and what we have are not fundamentally different."[9] In the second evolutionary scoop, "'Higher centers involved in emotional processing like the hippocampus and amygdala are a lot more elaborate in mice than in lizards." Finally, in the top scoop, ="humans have a giant, complex cortex. This is home to our thoughts and language." [10]

Brain Stem

The *brain stem*—in the first scoop at the top of the spine—manages processes like breathing, heartbeat, and other survival systems. We can simply trust this part of the brain to do its job without any attention or thought from the rest of the brain.

Limbic System

The brain parts in the second scoop—the center of the brain—process our emotions, memories, addictions, biological clock, hunger, and sensory information. It links the spinal cord to the cortex or thinking brain. (Its role in memory formation will be described in chapter 3.)

Looking at individual parts of the limbic system, the *thalamus* receives information from the senses, passing the neural package along to the hippocampus, where it begins its journey to become memories with whatever feeling tag that comes along. If we felt threatened, our *amygdalae* (we actually have two of them— one on either side of center) sends out the alert for fight or flight, short-circuiting that connection to the thinking brain; our survival is its main purpose. During chronic stress, the amygdalae trigger continual release of stress hormones, which can damage many parts of our brains and bodies. We can train the prefrontal cortex to calm the amygdalae so we can avoid being driven by fear. Wouldn't that be wonderful? That discussion will come in chapter 4. The *hypothalamus* takes care of our hormones and body clock, and the *nucleus accumbens*—our pleasure center—rounds out the group. They work together seamlessly and in milliseconds to coordinate our brain and body functions. [11]

Cerebral Cortex

This third and top "scoop" gives us our uniquely human capabilities. Our *cerebral cortex* houses 70 percent of the brain's synapses where most thinking actually happens. When people refer to our "gray matter," they are talking about this part of the brain. The cerebral cortex is only as deep as two dimes on top of each other, but the surface area is the size of an open newspaper. Its fissures and convolutions maximize the surface area; its folded surface is the part of the brain we often see in models and graphics. It has designated addresses for its various brain functions: vision (*occipital lobe*); problem solving, planning, conscience, and higher-level thinking

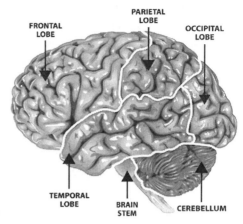

Figure 1. Sections of the Cerebral Cortex and Their Functions

(*frontal lobe*); spatial perception (*parietal lobe*); and sensory processing, touch, logic, math, language, and speech (*temporal lobe*).

If this part of the brain is damaged, it will not rebuild itself. Bike and other sports helmets are crucial to protect the brain.[12] Music, interpersonal communication, and many other kinds of activity use multiple locations together—exercising our brain.

Neuroscientists have drawn attention to the lasting effects of traumatic brain injuries in athletes and soldiers. After decades of brain-crippling concussions, brain health in this population is getting long overdue attention. NFL players and soldiers returning from military duty have had histories of debilitating mental health problems, leading to Alzheimer's and suicide, and this has been widely discussed and studied. Dr. Dorian McGavern suggests that minor trauma could contribute to the disease CTE (chronic traumatic encephalopathy), evidence of which has been found in autopsied brains of football players who committed suicide. Having one's "bell rung" used to mean, "Be tough and get back in the game." Now we know that a second concussion creates significantly more damage to the brain than the first. Coaches and athletic organizations are wisely insisting on assessments and brain recovery time after a player experiences a concussion.

Researchers are making progress, studying the causes, effects, and possible cures for concussions.[13] With information from fMRIs and SPECT scans, we can see what's going on in their brains, understand, and work on the problem. Studies in brain trauma recently revealed that applying antioxidants to the skull of mice immediately after a concussion reversed the damage to brain cells. Research will continue and hopefully help to preserve the lifetime brain health of our athletes and soldiers and others who suffer from traumatic brain injury. [14]

Cerebellum

Also called the "little brain," the *cerebellum* coordinates movements with the brain's motor cortex—the part of the brain that coordinates muscle movement. It takes over some processes when they have become automatic—like tying shoes, riding a bike, or even driving to work without actually paying attention to where we're going. Ever arrive and not remember the trip? Scary stuff!

Want to see your little brain at work? Simply fold your hands together. Notice which thumb is on top. Now, cross them the "wrong" way, putting the other thumb on top. It feels odd because your little brain is accustomed to doing it the other way. Over time and with practice, you can strengthen that specific neural package of muscle memory, teaching your little brain to be comfortable with the new connections.

Remember, creating new connections between the neurons in your brain gives you more choices of ways to accomplish tasks. Challenge your brain and spark new connections by trying to write your name with your non-dominant hand or count backwards or by intervals of more than one. The results are humbling at first, but it's the same process as when you learned all new things as a small child. Your brain adapts.

Doing things a new way requires your full attention, so your little brain goes on break and your "thinking brain" (see cerebral cortex, above) takes over, creating new pathways. Repeating new habits eventually creates new, stronger connections between cells. When they are well established, they will also become automatic and be saved in your little brain.

Corpus Callosum

Deep in the fissure between the right and left hemispheres, we find the *corpus callosum*, the passageway through which each hemisphere communicates with the other. Interesting fact about the corpus callosum—when we process humor, this four-inch-long collection of extremely dense synapses gets a major workout. The brain sends messages back and forth, gathering bits from all over the brain, so the joke or incident will make sense to us. Did you know that we can strengthen this left-right brain communication simply by repeatedly crossing the body's midline with our arms or legs? This can help you prepare for challenging mental tasks. Many educators include this as part of their students' daily routines.

Listening to and playing music exercises nearly every part of the brain, giving the corpus callosum a challenge, making it stronger. Dance to upbeat music for fun, and boost your brain and body health at the same time!

Neurons (or Brain Cells)

The brain's 100 billion *neurons* are linked together to send messages to make the mind and body work. They tell us when to eat, sleep, step, pick up something, or notice when something's wrong and needs our attention. A single neuron can send 250 to 2,500 nerve impulses per second. During a baby's development, all cells start out the same. But as they move or migrate, they take on the characteristics that are necessary for their ultimate destination and to accomplish the tasks that will await them there. They will specialize in processing language, visual functions, motor functions, or the executive functions in the prefrontal cortex.[15]

Dendrites

Each neuron's fingerlike extensions, or *dendrites*, gather information that comes from our senses or from other neurons. Each time we try something new, neurons activate, or "fire," together, creating a connection between them. Any given neuron can have thousands of connections to other brain cells and throughout the body. Each connection involves dendrites

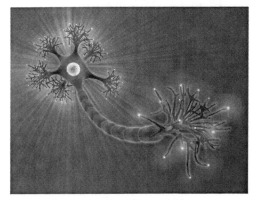

Figure 2. Dendrites, Neuron, and Myelinated Axon

and the spaces, or synapses, between them, through which the impulses travel, making it possible for the brain to do its work.

Axon

A brain cell can't do anything with information by itself. Communication is the key here, as it is between people. Attached to each brain cell, an electrically sensitive cord called the *axon* carries the message from one brain cell to the next one in line either in the brain or through the body. A single axon may have just a few branches or as many as 10,000, depending on the location and assignment. They may be just a fraction of an inch long or reach all the way from spine to toes. *Myelin*, a protective coating made from omega-3 fats wraps around each connection or axon. Think of an electrical cord with rubber insulation. This blanket of fat keeps the message on track and speeds the impulse along the pathway much faster than would happen in an unprotected axon. How fast? If you stub your toe, the pain message reaches the brain of a six-foot adult body in *two tenths of a second*. The axon also releases neurotransmitters, which either help the message along or stop it from passing through the synapse.

Synapses

Brain cells and axons do not actually touch each other. Much of the work that goes on in the brain takes place in the space between them, called *synapses*. Figure 3 shows the synapse with neurotransmitters that either speed up or slow down the impulse as it travels to the next cell. "The number of synapses may be as many as 1,000 trillion, or the number one followed by fifteen zeroes."[16] Trillion—what does that number mean, really? If we were to count one number per second, it would take 32,000 years to count to a trillion.

Oversimplifying what happens in each brain cell, national wellness speaker Jeff Haebig, PhD, uses

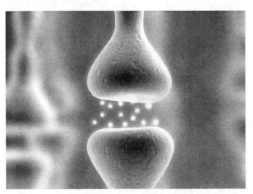

Figure 3. Synapses

rhythm, rhyme, and motion to describe how those bits of sensory information in the brain make our muscles move, create, and store memories or move our muscles:

- *Excite the dendrites,* the fingerlike extensions from each brain cell.
- *Turn on the neuron*: receiving new information from the dendrites wakes up or activates the brain cell, so it's ready to transmit information to the next one.
- *Fat on the axon*: myelin made from healthy fats coats the connection, or axon, much like an electrical cord. With that protection, the impulse speeds along the axon up to twelve times faster and keeps it from being scattered and lost along the way.
- *Peek through the synapse*: the space between brain cells where neurotransmitters either speed up or slow down the information, which must leap across that gap to link with another cell.[17]

It's Not All in Your Head

Now let's take a closer look at body/brain communication. The head holds the brain, but the mind involves the entire body and beyond. The central nervous system includes the spine and network of nerves, which extends throughout the body. They all work together to gather and transmit information to and from the brain.

We already know about eyes, ears, nose, tongue, and skin. The only way into the brain is through our senses. Another sensory contributor—our kinesthetic sense—is less recognized but very important. The entire body gets into the act. Each of our muscles and joints send messages directly to the *vestibular system*, which coordinates sensory input and passes it on to the brain. Most of us learn better when we activate our "muscle memory." This is why movement supports learning in a big way. Many people prefer hands-on learning for this reason.

My colleagues who are occupational therapists have helped me understand and appreciate the role of the *vestibular, proprioceptive,* and *ocular systems* in the learning and memory-making process. First, the vestibular system—located in the inner ear, not actually in the brain—coordinates the messages that come into the brain from our senses. It sends them on to the thalamus and midbrain for screening and processing. It works closely with the proprioceptive system—which connects the skeleton, muscles, and brain—to coordinate movement, balance, and sense of position in space. How does this happen? All of the body's muscles, bones, and tendons have receptors, which gather information about body movement, position, and balance. We use this network constantly for our awareness of the body's orientation as perceived by the eyes and brain which comprise the ocular system.

Once in the brain, this information goes to the part of the brain that controls movement. Repeating the action strengthens the connections between involved brain cells, eventually creating a habit. Once the cerebellum gets involved, that connection is ours for life.

So, there you have it. God's incredible creation within our heads, taking care of our lives. Surely appreciation and gratitude are in order!

Science may be able to explain how the systems of the brain work together, but it can't touch the vastness of this incredible creation of God. For that, we need poetry—such as this poem from Emily Dickinson.

The Brain Is Wider than the Sky

The brain is wider than the sky,
For, put them side by side,
The one the other will contain
With ease, and you beside.
The brain is deeper than the sea,
For, hold them, blue to blue,
The one the other will absorb,
As sponges, buckets do.
The brain is just the weight of God,
For, lift them, pound for pound,
And they will differ, if they do,
As syllable from sound.
—**Emily Dickinson** (1830–1886)

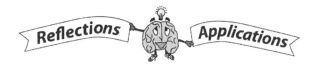

Reflection

Our God-created human brain is the most complex organism in the world. What part or brain function would you like to learn more about?

Application

1. How do you prefer to receive information? Is it easiest for you to read, listen, talk with others about it, write about it, or learn hands-on (kinesthetically)?

2. How are you most comfortable passing that information on to other people? Our favorite paths are often our most effective ones.

3. Teaching someone else what you've learned is a great way to lock the learning in your memory. Explain parts of brain function to someone else.

---

1   Michael S. Sweeney, *Brain—The Complete Mind: How It Develops, How It Works, and How to Keep It Sharp* (National Geographic, 2009), 13.

2   "The Neuroscience of Finding Your Lost Keys," Science Blog, March 21, 2013, http://scienceblog.com/61618/the-neuroscience-of-finding-your-lost-keys/#jVoGf5jeI1xGvoeO.99.

3   For more about educational kinesiology and the Brain Gym® exercises devised by Dr. Paul E. Dennison and Gail E. Dennison, visit www.braingym.org.

4   Nan Brien, "Great Beginnings: The First Years Last Forever," presentation, Wisconsin Council on Children and Families, 2000, 5.

5   Ibid., 4.

6   Caroline Leaf, "The Power Of The Brain, Part 1," video, https://www.youtube.com/watch?v=U38eiCOy0Ow.

7   Robert Klemko, "If You Give a Mouse a Concussion," *Sports Illustrated*, April 20, 2014, 43.

8   Sweeney, *Brain—The Complete Mind*, 10–14.

9   Kimberly Hiss, "The Beautiful Life of Your Brain," *Reader's Digest*, September 2014, 78-79.

10 Ibid.

11   Judith Horstman, *The Scientific American Day in the Life of Your Brain: A 24-Hour Long Journal of What's Happening in Your Brain as You Sleep, Dream, Wake Up, Eat, Work, Play, Fight, Love, Worry, Compete, Hope, and Make Important Decisions, Age, and Change* (Jossey-Bass, 2009), 4.

12   Brien, "Great Beginnings: The First Years Last Forever," 10.

13   Klemko, "If You Give a Mouse a Concussion," 43.

14   Ibid., 42.

15   Brien, "Great Beginnings: The First Years Last Forever," 8.

16   Sweeney, *Brain—The Complete Mind*, 13.

17   Adapted from Dr. Jeff Haebig's presentations. You can find more about his work on body/brain-based methods at www.wellnessquest.com.

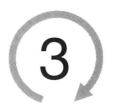

MEMORIES UNDER CONSTRUCTION

God gave us memory so that we might have roses in December.
—J. M. Barrie

A strange thing is memory, and hope; one looks backward,
and the other forward; one is of today, the other of yesterday.
Memory is history recorded in our brain, memory is a painter,
it paints pictures of the past and of the day.
—Grandma Moses (Anna Mary Robertson Moses)

What's her name? I've known her for years! Why can't I come up with her name? We may fear that we're losing our minds when we can't remember things that used to be right on the tip of our tongues. With advancing years, retrieval of memories slows down and we panic. Try not to worry. This doesn't mean you are seeing early signs of Alzheimer's. Give yourself a little more time and the memory will come back to you.

In this chapter, we will look at stages of memory formation, various types of memory, and their mechanics. The best part—and this may come as a surprise to you—is that our memory is renewable! As we learned in chapter 1, the brain's plasticity means that it changes constantly. It's up to us whether those changes are positive or negative. Memory processes might be the changes we notice the most. Unfortunately, stress makes any memory problems even worse. When we beat ourselves up for forgetting, we sabotage any chance of rescuing the elusive thought. Have you noticed that it pops into your head when you're relaxed and doing something completely unrelated to the topic you're trying to remember? Be gentle—don't try too hard. Take good care of your brain, and it will take good care of you.

With every year we live, we gather special memories of times with loved ones. With age, they become a rich treasure trove. Relationships are the only "possessions" we can keep with us—most of our stuff will be left behind. Memories are gifts, wrapped in our experiences and recorded through our senses. Here is one of my favorites from many years ago:

Our family tried camping while I was growing up—once. We went to Gooseberry Falls. Who knew Mom's fried chicken could be so tasty cold? Carrots and celery were sweeter than I remembered them tasting at home. The chocolate chips in her amazing cookies were still soft and gooey. My sister, brother, dad, and I made them disappear in a heartbeat.

Sleeping didn't go so well for me. I can remember being relieved when the night was over—maybe because I couldn't get comfortable with rocks under my thin sleeping bag and air mattress. After trying everything else, I ended up scrunched into the back seat of the car.

Dad came to check on me just before sunrise and gave me a favorite memory—still with me today. He wrapped his well-worn flannel shirt over my pajamas, and we went for a walk to the falls. He was a man of few words, but he comforted me with the gentle, loving strength of his arm around my shoulders. We snuggled together while beautiful colors danced in the sky. Rushing water made me forget there was any other place on Earth. Sitting close and wrapped in the smell of cherry pipe tobacco wafting from his favorite shirt, I felt warm, safe, and loved. Early morning birdcalls, the smell of damp dewy earth, and chilly early morning air all came together in this precious moment. His soft brown eyes sent love and peace my way with no need for words. His presence was enough — as long as he was with us.

The rest of the family teased me mercilessly for my camping cop-out. I don't remember us ever trying it again, which is our loss. My dad has been gone for many years, but every time I think of camping, I smile, feeling his love and presence. I'll treasure this memory and sensory bouquet forever.

Senses and Emotions

Everything entering the brain comes through our senses. The sensory message includes whatever emotion we are experiencing at the time. Our brain saves data as memories, with the emotion "tagging" along. When we are frightened or feel threatened, the brain jumps into action to keep us safe.

Neuroscientist Joseph W. LeDoux, a pioneer in the study of fear, gives us an example. When we see or hear something that might be a threat, our internal security system—the amygdala—sets off a chain of events to keep us safe and to fulfill its primary purpose. Fear generates neurochemical alarms in our brain and body, causing both physical and emotional reactions. Say we catch a glimpse of a face peeking in our window after dark. The amygdala's main job is to keep us safe.[1] Author Judith Horstman continues to describe LeDoux's process:

> The danger data race from the thalamus (the brain's receiver of information from the senses), to the amygdala through the cortex (the seat of reasoning that analyzes data) and/or the hippocampus (the memory and input center that compares the new information to past experiences), while your hypothalamus tells the adrenal and pituitary to pour cortisol and other stress hormones into the mix.
>
> Your amygdala is fast: it has its pistol out of the holster (enemy at the window!) before the thinking brain can chime in (it's your neighbor looking for her cat). It takes only twelve milliseconds for the thalamus to alert the amygdala, says LeDoux, who calls this emotional brain reaction the "low road." The "high road," or the trip through the thinking brain

and hippocampus, takes two or three times as long to process the input and send it back to the amygdala.[2]

The next day when we catch a glimpse of our neighbor or her cat, we may be surprised by a tightening in our bodies or another stress reaction. That's the body reacting to emotions recorded when we felt the threat on the low road.

Remembering that the brain's main priority is to keep us alive and safe, the feeling tag serves as a warning signal. If we felt threatened during the original experience, our personal homeland security system—the amygdala—will read that tag and send a warning to stay away the next time we encounter a similar situation. Cortisol shuts down our prefrontal cortex (PFC), or thinking brain. Without a working connection to our PFC, we run on pure emotion, often into trouble. If the feeling is warm and welcoming—like my time with Dad—I save it and reenter my memory of those special moments whenever I need to restore serenity.

Fast-forward to family life with our own children. When it was time for us to move, someone told us to fill our home with wonderful smells. Seriously? Baking bread helps sell our house? You bet! It worked! The first family that came offered more than our listed price! After the new owners had settled in, we talked with them about our aroma strategy. They said they felt right at home the minute they walked in the door—it must have been their own happy memories triggered by homey smells.

Turns out our sense of smell is the only one with a direct hookup to the hippocampus, the brain's memory coordination center. Every other sense takes longer to process before actually making a memory connection. Each of them must pass through the thalamus on their way.

We react emotionally and immediately to both positive and negative aromas stored in our memory banks. Think of a particular smell and the memories it triggers for you. Brats on the grill after a looong winter? First cut of the spring lawn? Fresh-baked anything? Real Christmas greenery? Newly sharpened pencils? Play dough? Or how about the smell of cleaning solutions in a hospital or school? A musty, dusty attic? Mucking out a barn? Immediate and emotional.

So now let's get specific about how this actually happens in our brains.

Memory Formation

The process of memory formation is complex. Something going wrong during any one of its four stages will leave us disconnected. We will look at all four stages: Acquisition, Consolidation, Retrieval, and Reconsolidation,[3] and how they work.

Stage 1: Acquisition

It all begins with our senses. Eyes, ears, nose, tongue, skin, and muscles take in the information. Neurons fire together creating a path "encoding" the information and bringing it into our short-term memory. The intensity of our attention determines the strength of the message. If we're distracted, the memory will be fuzzy and less likely to survive. When these neurons are activated, they form connections with other neurons all over the brain.

Have you heard, "When cells fire together they wire together?" That means two or more neurons become active at the same time. Scientists are now able to use special brain scans (fMRI) to help them actually see axons or connections between brain cells forming. If we were to watch someone's brain while they are motivated and trying something new, the scan would show a brand new trail blazing between two neurons when they "fire" together. This new connection is weak at first, but reinforced by a coating of myelin—like electrical tape—it protects the impulse and speeds it on its way.

Snow Path and Brain Connections

To illustrate the process of forming connections between brain cells, we can compare it to someone walking across freshly fallen snow, creating a path to a cabin in the woods. The first set of footsteps is disconnected, but with each pass, the gaps between the steps in the snow grow smaller. Eventually the path becomes solid and easy to find and follow. Over time, finding the way becomes automatic. With repeated exposure, some connections become more solid and permanent—like an interstate highway exchange, easy to access from many starting points.

Brain cells come in all shapes and sizes, some with thousands of extensions or dendrites. All brain cells originate from the same cell in the developing embryo. During their migration to their final brain destination, they miraculously take on the characteristics they will need to do their unique work in their assigned location. Let's take a closer look at the parts of the brain "assigned" to creating memories.

Limbic System: Memory Central

Revisiting the limbic system we introduced in chapter 2, we find it's the place where learning and creating memories begins. When sensory information enters the limbic system, which includes the thalamus, amygdala, and hippocampus, connections form between brain cells. We create these links through our experiences and strengthen them through repetition and practice.

Thalamus

The thalamus is the first stop and relay station for all sensory input except the things we smell. Scents have a direct route to the hippocampus, so memories associated with smells connect more quickly than any other senses. Everything else has to wait for the thalamus to send it forward.

Amygdala Guard

Next, it has to pass the "safety test" of Our brain's internal security system, the amygdala, which is the size and shape of an almond. It sits just above the hippocampus, where memories and feelings are processed. The amygdala monitors all incoming memories and experiences to guard the brain and body from possible threats. Survival is the brain's default concern. As "gatekeeper," the amygdala opens wide for comfort, joy, and peace, but blocks any threat before shipping that experience off to its ultimate storage spot in the brain.

Survival trumps both memory and new learning when the amygdala jumps into alert mode. The brain's ultimate assignment is to keep us alive, so other thinking functions go to the back burner. Now you know why it's hard to think straight when you're frightened. We will remember the fearful element of the experience as fear producing, but its content may escape us later.

Hippocampus

The hippocampus looks like a pair of horseshoes, which is how it got its name from the Greek language. Sensory information stops first at the amygdala to screen and register any emotional tags associated with a previous threat. If it's scary, the data is blocked and detoured while the sympathetic nervous system jumps to action releasing cortisol to give us extra energy and blood flow, so we can deal with the threat. Information that passes the "safety test" moves to the main part of the hippocampus—and our short-term memory.

Our ancestors found many ways to deal with emotions, some healthy and some not so much. Aromatherapy has relieved stress for centuries. It uses senses and calming memories to soothe the *central nervous system* (CNS). Shifting from *sympathetic* (fight or flight) to *parasympathetic* (rest and digest) mode helps every part of the body work better. It may use any combination of essential oils or candles, soft fabrics, soothing music, a hug, snuggling with a pet or favorite person, or massage to deliver the sensory smorgasbord. Nice to know we can take care of that naturally and on purpose!

Emotional Tags

Emotions highlight each of our learning experiences—either positively or negatively, as we discussed in chapter 2. Every memory is saved with whatever emotion we feel while it's encoding. If positive, it's filed with a "come back soon!" tag, gluing the memory so it will stick around. If we felt threatened during the experience, the amygdala flags the memory with a "danger" tag and will remind us to stay away when something similar approaches in the future.

Types of Memory Systems

While similar in having an emotional tag, our memories are built differently depending on their source and purpose. We will look at four memory systems: semantic (what), procedural (how), episodic (where), and automatic (now).[4]

What: Just the Facts

Memorizing facts through drill and practice—like the alphabet, math facts, or the periodic table of the elements—uses our declarative—also called semantic—memory. Add music or movements to make this learning or memories easier to recall later.

Where: Experiences and Personal Stories

Paying attention to our surroundings makes memory richer. Jesus loved using stories to help his followers, including us, learn important life lessons. Readers and audiences still respond to humorous stories, which help them learn and apply lessons. Why did I come into this room? What was I looking for? Ever walk into a room with some purpose in mind, only to completely forget what that purpose was?

"Whew! What a relief! Scientific proof that it's not me! I can blame it on the door!" I was at the kitchen sink and needed a spray bottle that I keep in the garage. I opened the door to the garage, and the dog sneaked out. I waited for her, and went back to get . . . what?

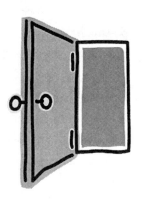

Researchers at the University of Notre Dame discovered that passing through a doorway triggers what's known as an *event boundary* in the mind. It IS all about the door! The thoughts and intentions from one environment are wiped clean when we enter a new one, clearing the slate for whatever awaits there. It's all about the brain's most important job—survival—keeping us ready for new surprises and vigilant for threats. Forgetting can be frustrating sometimes, for sure! But it's good to know it's not our age; it's that darn door!

How: Procedures

Many people prefer hands-on learning. It taps into multiple brain pathways, making the memory richer and easier to remember. My computer guru likes to ask me to "do it yourself" when he's trying to teach me a new process. He wisely insists muscle memory sticks longer than any other kind. I agree, in theory, but often still have trouble remembering exactly how to do it when I'm on my own. Guess I need more practice.

Now: Automatic Skills

We don't have to think about these skills when we do them on autopilot. We've already repeated those steps enough times—some say twenty-seven days; others say six weeks—until the brain takes over. Multitasking is an example of "now" memory, and it gets weaker as we get older. We choose only one or two parts of our experience to occupy the "main monitor" of our mind, but continue doing other things running "in the background." Without actually tuning in, we will probably not be able to remember doing them later. These "background functions" run on their own without access to the full collections of related facts. No wonder we make mistakes operating on "half a brain." Think of the huge risk drivers take when they make something else their primary focus—texting for example.

Stage 2: Consolidation

In this second stage, the brain chooses the memories worth the necessary brain space investment. Connections to existing memories strengthen the new information. It checks the newcomer against the entire collection of long-term memories already on file. Whatever matches gets to stick around; the rest is tossed.

This can happen in minutes, days, or much longer. The information that you encoded during the first stage must now pass the test to be saved. Consolidation preserves its spot in the brain's network. Applying the senses or associating it with something else helps make the memory stronger. Saying the person's name and matching it with an image that you'll remember might make it easier to recall later—saving us embarrassing moments.[5]

From Immediate to Short-Term/Working Memory

Sensory information enters *immediate memory* for milliseconds, then moves very quickly into *short-term* or *working memory*. There it gets three seconds to one minute to be used, repeated, or practiced.[6] We can say, write, or associate it with an image stored in another part of our brain in order to save it. Otherwise, we lose it to make room for whatever piles into our brain next.

Long-Term Memory

If the information matches something already stored in memory, it zips to *long-term memory*, which lasts from one minute to a lifetime, depending on how much it's used and the positive or negative emotion involved.

The brain constantly screens everything in our awareness, discarding what we don't need, making room for more important things—always trying to keep us safe, which is job number one. Most of what we encounter doesn't stick, because we wouldn't have room to store it all! In this case, forgetting is a very good thing. If it relates to what we already have chosen to save, it sticks like Velcro hook-and-loop closures. If it's completely new to us, it slides away as if on Teflon nonstick coating.

The brain isn't particularly loyal to new bits of information. Disconnected pieces are tossed—usually while we are in a deep sleep—to make room for more "valuable" bits of information. Intentionally focusing on them can give them staying power. Once they earn the transfer to long-term memory, they will be saved, or "consolidated," and remain at the appropriate combination of brain addresses until we bring them back to our "main monitor." Our choices can either help or hinder that process.

Consolidation Happens Differently for Each Type of Memory

While we're asleep, "what" (semantic) and "where" (location) or "when" (episodic) information is promoted to long-term memory. Studies show a nap often makes it easier to remember what we've learned. A woman in one of my seminars told me about her daughter, a premed student. She always plans a forty-five-minute nap break into her study sessions. Adding rest for her brain has made a big difference in the effectiveness of her learning. Her naps apparently don't interfere with falling asleep at the end of the day. Ah, to be young!

Practice, repetition, and adding sensory cues support consolidation of our "how," or procedural, memories. For example, keyboard skills take lots of eye/hand focus while learning, but they become automatic when used regularly. Playing an instrument may be a struggle at first, testing the patience of the friends and family who can't escape when we're learning. Over time, it becomes easier for us and more fun for others.

The next stage can be frustrating if we are impatient with our brains.

Stage 3: Retrieval

This stage involves bringing memories back up onto our "main monitor." Trying to recall information, especially under pressure, is a challenge as we grow older. The brain must reactivate the pattern created the last time we accessed the memory. Interruptions can easily sidetrack our thinking. Frustrating!

Recalling familiar information happens in the blink of an eye. The system automatically returns to friends' phone numbers or passwords we use every day. Recognizing a face begins by processing the visual image, then checks to see if the person is familiar to us—all in less than a second. Coming up with a name we haven't used in a while may be tougher with age. It happens to all of us.

Complex recall takes more work. Say someone has asked you for driving directions to a restaurant you've recommended to them or even another town. First, you may mentally retrace the route you followed to get there yourself. If it's been awhile, you may need to refresh your memory by consulting a map or an online app. Then you would choose how to share the route with your friend so they will be able to follow the directions while driving. Some people just tell them the directions; others draw a map, write in words or a text, or send a link. This all takes time and focus.

Add the pressure we place on ourselves when we can't retrieve a name or other bit of information, and the brain simply locks up. The amygdala interprets our intense effort as stress and triggers release of cortisol, which stops the process cold. "It's right on the tip of my tongue . . . ." It often comes back to us when we ease up on ourselves, think of something else, or relax the brain. My brain usually completes the cycle when I'm laughing with another friend. When the light goes on, I tell them about it, and our laughter takes off again. Yep. It happens to everyone.

Patience, gentleness, and an active sense of humor can actually help. Judgment, criticism, and high expectations can trigger our fearful amygdala, quickly shutting down whatever memory we are able to access. Take it easy, and enjoy the journey.

Next, we'll look at actually changing our memories! Interesting concept!

Stage 4: Reconsolidation

Ever wonder why people who witnessed the same event may recall it differently? It's all about brain mechanics. Did you know we change our memories each time we recall them? New information, new feelings, or being in a different place—literally and figuratively—add new dimensions to our memory package. Thoughts, feelings, and other bits of information recently stored as memories can cause us to change or edit details or even forget some parts of the event. Think about the way a woman recalls the childbirth experience and how this memory changes over time. Her emotions give the labor and delivery memory some stability, but hormones released during birth make her mercifully forget some of the intensity of that memory and replace it with overwhelming love.

Emotion Revises Memories

Another odd thing about memories: Emotion partners along with them, but the brain also revises them with every recall. Each of us builds our own "filter" through which we choose to interpret our sensory input. We choose to notice and hold on to different aspects of each event depending on the emotions we experienced at the time. We couldn't possibly remember everything in our environment, so our brain selects those parts, which have meaning for us. That filter determines what we save as memories.

Research explains differences in memories between people who shared the same experiences. Siblings may seem to have grown up in completely different families based on their memories. Our filters are fluid, changing with new learning and interpretations of our experiences. Each time we review what we remember, we add new information and emotion, editing the memory package so it fits our current filters. Actually, going back, recalling memories, telling stories, and creating and going through scrapbooks, digital photo books, and videos can keep our memory machinery sharp!

Keeping a visual reminder of special memories can keep them fresh—like reconnecting with old friends. With those tools, our relationships may be able to pick up right where they left off, letting the years fall away since they were created.

Your Brain—a Renewable Resource

Remember the warning, "You can't teach an old dog new tricks?" Now we know the hippocampus—where memories are generated—is plastic, meaning that it's changeable over time. With the right input and challenges, we can choose to keep it growing and changing throughout our lives. Very good news!

Studies conducted in the new field of adult neurogenesis bring both encouragement and a warning. Rockefeller University's Elizabeth Gould's research outcomes were described in *Scientific American*: "Thousands of new cells are generated in the adult brain every day, particularly in the hippocampus, a structure involved in learning and memory. Within a couple of weeks, most of these newborn neurons will die, unless the animal is challenged to learn something new. Learning—especially that involving a great deal of effort—can keep these new neurons alive."[7]

So although our hippocampus generates thousands of new cells a day, these cells fade if they're not challenged, but they're ours to keep if we give them a good workout. They are not "vested" until they get a major workout. Without a "brain boost," they're gone in a couple of weeks.

We all know that mental changes happen, and we are wise to notice them and take care of our brains accordingly. The good news—not all the changes are negative. As mentioned in the introduction, you'll find the "Bless the Boost" and "Fight the Fade" sections at the close of each of the four parts of Max Your Mind. "Bless the Boost" will be your opportunity to celebrate those brain skills that stay the same or improve with age. "Fight the Fade" will acknowledge and help you deal with those that decline, offering strategies to help you make the most of your mind. Give them a try to ease your frustration with the changes and reduce their impact on your life. Thanks for hanging in there so far, and treasure your memories!

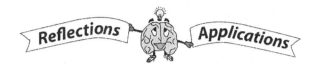

Reflection

Have you ever forgotten why you came into a room? Are you able to laugh about it without judging yourself or panicking about losing your mind?

Application

1. How do you deal with event boundary? What helps you keep your intention in mind when moving from one room to another?

2. Recall an event that seems different to you now than when it first happened. Discuss the changes in this memory package with another person who shared the original experience with you.

3. Can you recall your brain going blank when you were fearful or upset? Think about your amygdala—your internal security system—and the "protection" it provides. Sometimes we might want to let our executive function—the prefrontal cortex—calm it down so we will be able to function.

---

1   Horstman, *The Scientific American Day in the Life of Your Brain*, 140.
2   Ibid., 141–42.
3   Nelson with Gilbert, *Achieving Optimal Memory*, 16–25.
4   Ibid.
5   Ibid., 18.
6   Ashish Ranpura, Brain Connection website, http://brainconnection.positscience. com (2007).
7   Key concepts compiled by the editors of *Scientific American* to introduce "Saving New Brain Cells" by Tracy J. Shors, *Scientific American*, March 2009, 46.

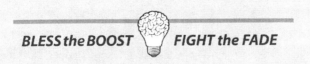

BLESS the BOOST   FIGHT the FADE

Bless the Boost and Fight the Fade: Your Brain

Bless the Boost

Let's look more closely at some of the mental skills that either improve or stay the same as we grow older:

- Language: Our personal word bank expands with each experience we encounter and each book we read. An average adult native speaker's vocabulary includes about 20,000 words with avid readers much higher. Being able to communicate our thoughts using this vast store of words is a definite benefit. Keep reading and talking with friends about what you've read. Doing so can only help build our brains!

- Focusing: Being able to pay attention to a task or story doesn't decline, and may improve with maturity. Experience makes it easier for us to know what's important and screen out distractions.

- Automatic skills: Over the years, we have committed many processes to memory. Once those brain cells are saved in long-term memory, they're ours to keep.

- Planning: We have trained our brains to plan many activities, small and large, and considered many potential outcomes—often through making our own mistakes. This accumulated information is available to help us avoid problems in the present and future.

Fight the Fade

The passing years have probably highlighted a "fade" or two in our mental prowess. Knowing we're not alone can be comforting, but here are some ways to deal with it:

- Working or short-term memory: Trying to remember the seven digits of a phone number, a name, or another bit of information long enough to use it can be frustrating—and it gets worse with age. Involve your senses to give it staying power. Try putting it to music, tying it to an image in your head, writing it down, or speaking it out loud so you can hear it.

- Remembering details: When we form a memory at an event or a talk, it's easier to lose some of the details than it used to be. Sometimes it helps to pay extra close attention during the input stage by writing something down or even taking a photo. Revisiting the experience through the words or image might bring it back with more clarity.

- Word retrieval: When the words—or name—just won't come, cut yourself some slack. Give yourself some extra time to think, and if that doesn't help, fess up. Chances are, the people you're with will understand and possibly laugh about it with you. Laughing together is a great way to build relationships. Whatever you do, don't panic or judge yourself. That's a sure way to make the situation worse.

- Reaction time: This can be a safety issue. As we grow older, it may take us a bit longer to react and respond to situations. Keeping loose rugs and clutter off the floor can prevent falls at this stage of our life. Vigilance in driving requires careful attention to both sides of the vehicle in addition to the forward view. Focus on only one thing at a time. Multitasking can create problems that could be easily avoided.

Part II
THE BODY

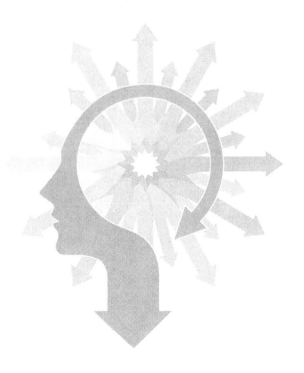

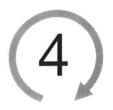

YOUR BODY
AS STRESS BUSTER

It's not stress that kills us; it is our reaction to it.
—Hans Selye

The brain gives the heart its sight; the heart gives the brain its vision.
—Rob Kall

The brain can spin into a frenzy, rehashing past events we can't change and worrying about future challenges that probably won't happen. Over time, that often leads to preventable illness. With body and brain working together, we will feel more peaceful and live lives that are more satisfying. Our minds and bodies let us know when something's not working—if we pay attention. We can avoid these problems by noticing and responding to the body's signals. In this chapter, we will look at the body's reaction to stress, consider strategies for dealing with it, and close with another personal story. Stress is unavoidable, but it doesn't have to take us down.

Stress Defined

Without any stress, we wouldn't be able to function. Our minds and bodies need a certain amount of stress in order to get us out of bed in the morning. However, too much, for too long, can and does make us sick.

The American Institute of Stress has a popular definition of stress that rings true for many of us. They say it's "a condition or feeling experienced when a person perceives that demands exceed the personal and social resources the individual is able to mobilize." [1] They list fifty common signs of stress, including "frequent headaches, jaw clenching or pain, gritting, grinding teeth." [2] I won't list them all, but you can probably create your own list from personal experience.

They describe both acute and chronic stress. When we experience a quick burst of cortisol during acute stress (fight or flight), our body's metabolism is able to return to normal in about ninety minutes. During chronic, everyday stress—financial, relationship, and work—we stop noticing the signs. [3] The body doesn't get a chance to recover, and the cortisol builds up over time. That accumulation of cortisol can cause health issues like heart disease, stroke, high blood pressure, depression, and sleep disorders. Preventing these effects is worth our attention.

As you know very well by now, the brain's main mission is to keep us alive. It sees everything else as secondary. When we're anxious or worried, it triggers the release of cortisol, which revs up our autonomic nervous system—including brain, spinal cord, and nerves throughout the body. We don't realize that cortisol has taken control of the body. Survival becomes more important than thinking clearly or remembering important lessons we may have learned in the past.

When we're feeling stress, the brain senses a threat and activates survival action, which is experienced as "fight or flight" mode. It signals the release of cortisol to keep us alive. To help us face the threat, cortisol speeds up our heartbeat and breathing and gives our muscles an added boost. That process gives us what we need to survive. But, without a break from stress, cortisol becomes toxic to our bodies—like an acid dump.

Our minds and bodies let us know when something's not working; we must pay attention and respond to signals like fatigue, headaches, and anxiety. Healthy choices keep the body and mind working at their best. Breathing can get us started.

Using Breath to Switch from Stress to Rest and Digest

Tapping into our breath can switch our body's nervous system from fight or flight (our *sympathetic nervous system,* or SNS) to rest and digest (our *parasympathetic nervous system*, or PNS). During stress, our SNS acts like a gas pedal in a car. The heart beats faster, breathing speeds up and gets shallower, and our bodies get ready for action to keep us safe. Anxiety follows, and our ability to think clearly shuts down.

Our breath can bring us back to peace. It flips the switch, activating our PNS, which cleanses the body and draws in the fresh oxygen our brain needs to function. Since the breath is part of the ramping up, we can choose to use it to help calm things back down.

Deep breathing activates the *vagus nerve*, which extends from the brain all the way to the intestines. It sends messages between heart, brain, and digestive system. The PNS acts like a brake, slowing our heart rate and giving the body a chance to calm and heal itself. Simply directing attention to our incoming and outgoing breath brings our focus inside and into the present moment, away from the past or future issue that caused the shift to guilt or panic.

On-purpose breathing seems to help many people calm their busy minds. Experiment with this pattern for five cycles:

- Inhale to a count of five, expanding your belly but keeping shoulders relaxed.
- Pause for two counts.
- Exhale for five, watching your belly recede.
- Let your body naturally begin the next inhale.

You may have felt a bit more relaxed after your experiment. If that didn't happen for you, repeat the breathing exercise three times, and then breathe normally. It may take some practice. Belly breathing is a tool that makes use of the complete capacity of our lungs. Opening them up all the way from the bottom to the top allows space for their important work: filling the blood with oxygen so it can travel and nourish the brain and body. Who knew that the simple act of tuning into our ever-present breath could calm the body's nervous system?

Any time we draw our attention inside our bodies, the stressors outside—past and future—have less impact on our thoughts and body systems. With practice, we can learn to activate our PNS to calm us and restore nurturing peace. It may take some time to learn how to calm ourselves, but the health and mental benefits will be well worth the effort.

The Institute of Heart Math teaches another strategy they call the Quick Coherence Technique. It helps body, brain, and breath to calm our nervous system and counteract the effects of cortisol on our bodies. The body's systems work better in coherence with each other. The following steps are excerpted from one of their pamphlets:

The Steps of the Quick Coherence Technique
1. Heart Focus: Focus your attention on the area around your heart.
2. Heart-Focused Breathing: Maintain your heart focus and, while breathing, imagine that your breath is flowing in and out through the heart area. Breathe casually, just a little deeper than normal.
3. Heart Feeling: Recall a positive feeling and make a sincere attempt to relive that feeling. You can recall a time when you felt appreciation or care for someone or something and attempt to re-experience that feeling. Once you have found a positive feeling, sustain it by continuing with the Quick Coherence steps: heart focus, heart-focused breathing, heart feeling.[4]

Choosing to breathe this way can improve our ability to think clearly, help our bodies heal, and allow our brains and bodies to work the way God designed them.

Each of us has our own package of stressors, but caring for ill family members seems to be at the top of the intensity chart. Sometimes the best thing we can do for relief is to go to bed at night. A friend who cares for her ailing mother says she looks forward to sleep as the best part of her day. Many mature "sandwich generation" folks who are caring for both children and parents can understand her situation. (More on this in chapter 13.) While our body rests, the brain stays busy clearing toxins and getting us ready for another day.

Sleep

Parts of the brain restrict incoming information while we sleep; giving other parts a chance to do their "second shift" job. Without deep sleep, we begin the next day with yesterday's clutter still grabbing for our attention. After short-sleep nights, my brain's "filing cabinet" feels as cluttered as the top of my desk sometimes looks.

A good night's sleep can make all the difference in our overall mood. Why do many of us get impatient and cranky when our brains don't get enough deep sleep? It's simple. While we're sleeping, the brain's "night crew" sorts and files all the experiences and information we've packed in during the day, saving and filing the important stuff and discarding the rest.[5]

While we are sleeping, the brain's tiny glial cells are busy removing toxins—neural waste from our brains. Dr. Maiken Neidergaard, co-director of the University of Rochester Medical Center for Translational Neuromedicine, published findings of a 2012 study. She dubbed this ". . . the 'Glymphatic system' because it acts like the body's lymphatic system but is managed by brain cells known as glial cells. The Glymphatic system clears away toxins or waste products that could be responsible for brain diseases, such as Alzheimer's disease and other neurological disorders."[6] Getting the deep sleep we need protects our healthy brains.

You might consider these tips from the National Sleep Foundation if you're struggling with insomnia:

1. Pay attention to light and your sleep patterns.
   - Manage your light exposure, and your body's circadian rhythms will adjust to your chosen schedule.
   - Sunlight or artificial light in the morning will wake up your brain.
   - Keeping lights dim before bed will let your brain prepare to fall asleep.
2. Avoid heavy food, alcohol, and nicotine.
   - Alcohol may make you feel sleepy, but when the effects wear off, it can leave you wide awake in the middle of the night.
   - Cigarettes and caffeine[7] can disrupt sleep.

- Eating big or spicy meals within two to three hours of going to bed can keep your digestive system too busy to relax for sleep.

3. Wind down gradually before bed.
   - Help your brain and body shift into sleep mode.
   - Spend the last hour before bed engaged in a calming activity such as reading or taking a warm bath.
4. Choose a different place to relax if you have trouble sleeping.
   - Train your brain to associate your bed with only sleep or sex.
   - Keep electronics out of the bedroom because their lights stimulate the brain.[8]

Knowing that sleep is important sometimes isn't enough. As we get older, many of us struggle to get the sleep we need. Here are some additional things to consider if that describes you.

Consistent Sleep Routines

During seasonal changes, many folks struggle with fatigue. Our bodies' circadian rhythms—or body clocks—take a few days to reset when we switch to and from Daylight Savings Time. Traveling through time zones and getting up with children or aging parents also compromise consistent zzzz's. When it's possible, a consistent sleep routine will help all the body's systems work better.

Pump It Up Early

Exercise has proven to help in our sleep department.[9] Walking, Pilates, and yoga keep my fibromyalgia under control most days. When I don't stretch, my body protests. On days when I don't get enough exercise, particularly outdoors, I have trouble falling asleep. When the weather allows, a brisk walk outdoors seems to help. A good workout pumps oxygen and nutrients to my body's cells, which then seem happier—provided I don't overdo it. If I exercise too close to bedtime, I can't wind down. Pumping it up earlier in the day gives my heart enough time to return to its comfortable resting rate. (More on this in chapter 6.)

Gratitude Grooms the Brain for Rest

Urgency for sleep creates counterproductive stress. When I'm anticipating a trip or important event the next day, I can count on waking up in the middle of the night. Then the chatter begins: *Get back to sleep! You don't have much time . . . sleep fast!* If you've ever experienced that, try shifting your focus: *I'm glad at least I'm getting some rest.*

Chiding myself for not falling asleep only makes it worse. After twenty minutes of struggling to fall asleep, a change of scene might help. I like to get up and go into another room. Focusing on a magazine, book, or piece of music helps clear my head and makes me drowsy enough for some real rest.

When regrets or worries kidnap the mind, keeping us from restful sleep, a shift to appreciation can calm the brain and heart. Updating my gratitude list before climbing into bed is one of my favorite habits. (You'll find more on gratitude in chapter 9.)

It creates calm and allows me to slip into rest mode.

One Muscle at a Time

Progressive muscle relaxation gives my body the message that it's time to let go. Paying attention to our breath makes it even more effective. Lying flat in bed, it's easy to scrunch up one set of muscles—say the head and face—inhale to a count of five, then let everything completely relax on the exhale, also to a count of five. Moving down the body working one set at a time lets the brain know it's time for rest. After relaxing your toes, let your body feel heavy and sink into the bed. Take one more deep breath and let go of your day.

Waking up naturally refreshed is priceless. The new day has so much to offer when we can be present and able to enjoy its blessings. Creating your own sleep routine can be challenging, but when it becomes a habit, your body and brain will thank you.

Cancer Care—Stress and Body Issues

Sometimes our bodies create rather than resolve stress. In October 2010, mine gave me a good reason to practice stress management. Changing clothes between yoga and golf that Friday morning, I discovered dimpling and felt a lump in my left breast. All heat left my body as a wave of questions washed over me.

Now what? Maybe it's nothing. Who should I call? What should I do? My April mammogram was clear. How could this happen?

When I couldn't think straight, I called my friend Diann Greener. She had been through this. After a few calls to clinics, my husband, Bob, and I decided to go ahead and keep our tee time. Sitting home worrying wouldn't make the wait any easier. I tried to concentrate on hitting the golf ball and keeping it out of patches of fallen leaves.

Everything looked the same, but it wasn't for me! How could ordinary life go on when mine was crashing down?

The nurse practitioner saw me that afternoon and got the ball rolling for my diagnosis and treatment. We met with the surgeon after a diagnostic mammogram and ultrasound. The diagnosis was invasive ductal carcinoma of the breast—the most common and treatable breast cancer. He said, "I have encouraging news— if there is a good cancer, this is it." Then why didn't I feel better?

Diann offered to be my cancer coach. She had walked this path and told me she wanted to help someone else through the journey. I was immensely grateful for her wisdom and experience! We talked about posting the story on a care site. That's a very personal decision, but I agreed to share the story to invite prayer support. God knew exactly what we needed and wanted. Being open to prayer and accepting help from friends, relatives, and my Peace Lutheran Small Group brought me peace and love during those tough times.

We scheduled surgery for my birthday. Not my first choice, but I couldn't wait to get the cancer out of my body; good thing I didn't know it would take more than once. Diann came to be with us before each one. She had given her surgical team a prayer she prayed before her procedure, and she offered it to me for my team. I was thankful my surgeon was also willing to pray that prayer for me.

Many thoughts surged through my head anticipating surgery that I knew would compromise my healing and outcomes. I listened several times to Diann's meditation CD before each surgery to prepare my own body, mind, and spirit for the experience. Relaxation wasn't possible in the pre-op bay, but I tried deep breathing and came prepared with iPod music. All the efficient professional activity going on around me blocked out the music. Knowing prayer would be part of my procedure helped me to trust the outcome to God. Praise God, I was cancer free—"No Evidence of Disease" (NED) after the third surgery. The next step was scheduling chemotherapy and radiation to keep it from coming back.

While we waited for my chemotherapy, Bob's routine checkup revealed lung cancer in his right lung. Never a smoker, lung cancer had made surgical removal of the lower lobe of his left lung necessary in 2009. "Take a deep breath, we can get through this . . ." After a second opinion, we started preparing physically and emotionally to become a dual chemotherapy household. He put his treatments off for a couple of months so he would be able to better help with my care. Our oncologist scheduled our chemo appointments so we wouldn't both hit "nadir"—the physical low point in the cycle—at the same time. We were able to take turns as caregiver and patient. Tragic? Comical? It was both, but God kept our sense of humor active through those months.

I dreaded losing my hair. When it started falling out, Diann said, "We might as well make it a celebration!" I didn't feel much like celebrating, but she was right. Sharing it lightened the load somehow. Laughter and supportive friends are amazing stress reducers. Kathy and Diann went with me to pick out wigs. Dar styled my wigs and later brought her salon to my home. Brave friends I called my "shearing angels" came to bring love and laughter to the occasion. They chose the highlighted "party" wig for me to wear that evening. Then Nancy, Kathy G., Kathy R., Diann, Char, and I went out for dinner. Somehow, even the food tasted good to me. Hooray, no metal taste!

That evening, they kept me focused on the precious present. We laughed a lot. Their prayers and presence stayed with Bob and me throughout the cancer journey. They showed us God's love in a very special way—one step at a time.

However, the challenges wouldn't stop! A few weeks later while taking a shower, I slipped and fell, crushing my right elbow. My orthopedic surgeon implanted a post at the top of my radius bone. Going into surgery again crushed my spirit, but the surgeon couldn't help with that—it was another opportunity to practice trust. I needed lots of help, and it came in the form of buckets of love and laughter.

The surgeon said he didn't expect me to regain full range of motion. He and my oncologist chose to suspend my chemotherapy while my elbow healed. Relieved for the break from chemo, I found new energy and determination to follow my physical therapist's treatment plan and home exercises. Months later, both my physical therapist and orthopedic surgeon were amazed that following the prescribed treatment plan, I had indeed restored full range of motion in that elbow. God's blessings are new each and every day.

Bob's friends came to pick him up and sit with him through his chemotherapy appointments. The nurses commented about all the laughter coming from his treatment room. At home, my attempts to be Bob's one-armed caregiver brought more tragic/comical scenes, but no more injuries, Praise God!

Looking back at these struggles, I think chemobrain was the worst. Having studied the brain for most of my life, I became very frustrated when mine stopped working the way it used to—before chemo. Several resources confirmed other cancer survivors' struggle with chemobrain. It's true, and it's debilitating! For some patients, it continues for *years* after treatment stops.

Reading was hard. I couldn't stay with a train of thought active long enough to follow the plot. Distractions had my mind jumping from one thought to another without finishing any one of them. My short-term memory was shockingly shorter and less accurate. I had trouble remembering where I put things and more problems trying to find them again. Details escaped my memory. Coming up with the right word became an arduous task. Family and friends patiently waited while I completed my internal word search. I struggled to dig my way through the dense fog wrapped around my brain. Turning to my standbys, writing and exercise, made it somewhat easier for me.

Journaling helped. Writing gave my brain another shot at forming memories about events and our situations. I brought my laptop to appointments so I could remember doctors' answers to our questions and their recommendations. We hadn't seen anyone use a personal laptop for notes, but someone had to be the first.

Exercise through the YMCA's LIVESTRONG program helped both of us focus on positive activity. We met delightful new friends and enjoyed the workout tailored to our physical levels. Skype and in-person family visits refilled our joy supply.

Returning via photos and video to Kananaskis County in the Canadian Rockies became my favorite meditation "vacation" from our bleak winter. I had spoken at a special education conference there a few days before discovering the lump. After my presentations, I had hiked up to a mountain meadow and soaked up its remote and inviting freshness. A scout troop passed the meadow, making their way back down the path after their day hike. They stopped to talk with me. Their enthusiasm and stories about their discoveries brightened that day as well as my "return visits" from my recliner. My souvenir Canada Bear super-soft sweatshirt completed the sensory picture whenever I needed to remind myself of joy and peace. It was a blessing and a memory gift I will treasure.

Complementary therapies helped me deal with pain, muscle issues, and nausea. Weekly acupuncture helped my upset stomach. My muscles released their tension during my massages. My chiropractor helped me monitor changes and removed the kinks from all my recliner time. Healing touch kept energy moving through my body so it could heal itself.

Cancer sparks so much stress and cortisol; we did what we could to stay upbeat. At four years from my diagnosis, I'm still NED, but also still notice shades of processing problems, but mental exercise—like writing a book—seems to help me move forward.

Some strong sensations from those difficult days remain as strong memories:

- While the chemo dripped into my port, I felt my life's energy surge from my body.
- Long hours at home became a challenge; the clock's pendulum kept me company.
- My Heart Math Emwave monitor helped me to focus on the present moment and avoid rushing ahead to worries about the future.
- Baking a batch of cookies took all day—with twenty-minute breaks between steps to restore my energy.
- I remember being thrilled to finally have the energy I needed to make the bed!

- Gratitude for many little things comes much easier after that experience.

Continuing my writing and speaking with a modified schedule helped me feel mentally alive. Building Baby's Brain and Music and the Brain classes gave my spirit a boost, but I allowed several days afterwards to recover my energy. Now I can smile at my gratitude for radio instead of TV interviews, sitting in my home office, bald as a baby's behind.

Stress management practice was one of the positive outcomes from our cancer experience. We also learned how to move away from regrets and worries and focus on the present moment's gifts. Facing serious illness and being with many others who are dealing with worse challenges gives us a new perspective. For that, I will always be grateful.

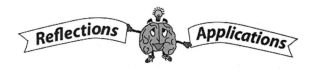

Reflection

Pause to consider and be thankful for each part of your body that is working properly. What an amazing creation!

Application

1. How do your mind, body, and spirit respond to focused breathing? Are the centering exercises helpful for your mental and emotional well-being?
2. Choose a person, place, or experience that you can focus on in order to bring your mind into peace and serenity. Take three deep belly breaths with this loving image in your mind. Practice this daily, and notice if it helps you with stress.
3. Try journaling to clarify your own thoughts and feelings, then revisit what you've written a month later to notice if the insights you wrote are helpful over time.

1   You can find this definition and other useful information about stress at The American Institute of Stress website, http://www.stress.org/daily-life/.

2   The American Institute of Stress, "50 Common Signs and Symptoms of Stress," http://www.stress.org/stress-effects/#sthash.5BYq9Fjt.dpuf.

3   The American Institute of Stress, "Definitions," http://www.stress.org/daily-life/

4   *Reducing Stress and Creating Better Health* (HeartMath LLC, Boulder Creek, CA). This pamphlet can be accessed at http://www.heartmath.com/wp-content/uploads/2014/04/client_edu.pdf.

5   Horstman, *The Scientific American Day in the Life of Your Brain*, 174–176.

6   Catharine Paddock, "Sleep Helps 'Detox' Your Brain," The Center for Sleep Medicine, http://www.chicagosleepstudy.com/sleep_helps_detox_your_brain.html.

7   National Sleep Foundation, "Caffeine and Sleep," article reviewed by Dr. Greg Belenky, http://sleepfoundation.org/sleep-topics/caffeine-and-sleep.

8   National Sleep Foundation, "Healthy Sleep Tips," http://sleepfoundation.org/sleep-tools-tips/healthy-sleep-tips/page/0%2C1.

9   Barbara Phillips, "Ask the Expert: Can Exercise Help with Excessive Sleepiness?" February 25, 2013, National Sleep Foundation website, http://sleepfoundation.org/ask-the-expert/can-exercise-help-excessive-sleepiness.

INPUT FOR OUTPUT

Food is medicine. It is the most powerful tool we have to combat chronic disease.
—Mark Hyman [1]

*The doctor of the future will give no medicine, but will interest his patients
in the care of the human frame, a proper diet, and preventing disease.*
—Thomas Edison

E ver wonder how we know when we need to eat? Our brain has a special control section at the base of the brain (referred to as the "first scoop" in chapter 2) which keeps track of blood levels of glucose, insulin, and the hormones *ghrelin* and *leptin* to make sure the body is getting enough calories and nutrients. Its technical name and location is the *arcuate nucleus*, within the hypothalamus. When these nutrients reach low levels, this part of the brain jumps into action. According to *The Scientific American Day in the Life of Your Brain:*

The arcuate nucleus regulates your appetite by counting calories for you—sort of. It monitors your blood levels of glucose and insulin and the hormones ghrelin and leptin to see if your body has enough calories and nutrients. Ghrelin, produced in cells lining the stomach, stimulates appetite: ghrelin levels rise before meals and fade after you've eaten. Its counterpart, the hormone leptin (mostly produced from fat tissue), puts the brakes on appetite after you've eaten—most of the time . . . . The arcuate nucleus adjusts your appetite, and some of its neurons can upset all those diet plans. They contain a substance, neuropeptide Y (NPY) that influences hunger. When activated, these neurons can stimulate what amounts to eating binges that empty your fridge and pack on the pounds.[2]

So now we know where to send the blame.

The problems begin when we live to eat rather than eating to live. "It's thought that two brain mechanisms control our food intake. The hypothalamus tells us when we need to eat to maintain our body weight "set point," much like a thermostat set on a specific temperature. Other brain centers such as the dopamine reward system control our desire to eat. When you covet a bowl of chocolate ice cream after dinner—a food that you don't *need* to eat but *want* to eat—it's your dopamine reward system getting excited."[3]

Dopamine goes to the brain's reward center, working like an addiction. No wonder why so many of us struggle with weight problems! Knowing that doesn't make maintaining a healthy weight any easier, but understanding may help us find ways to deal with the issue.

Positive Choices for the Brain

Our amazing brain, that three-pound bundle of neurons and synapses between our ears, needs a steady supply of fuel to accomplish the 400 trillion processes it completes every second.[4] It depends on our choices—what we eat and drink — for its input. It can't store the glucose it needs to work. Our circulatory system is the only source for its fuel.

The brain is 80 percent water, and uses 25 percent of the body's energy to do its important work. The food and drink we choose to ingest can make or break the quality of the supply of nutrients the brain is able to use. Healthy choices will keep the brain's fuel supply coming, making it easier for us to think clearly and be satisfied with our brain's "output."

Our Bodies, God's Gift

According to Mark Hyman, one author of *The Daniel Plan*, "The scriptures teach us how to live and love fully. But somehow, we skip over the parts that instruct us to honor the vessel of the Holy Spirit, our body. Being in a food coma from eating sugar and junk food, having your brain chemistry hijacked by hyper-processed, hyper-palatable, hyper-addictive foods prevents you from fully inhabiting your body and your mind. If the food you are eating is making you sick and unfocused and makes you so sluggish that if you happen to get the urge to exercise, you instead lie down until it goes away, living a fully engaged and God-honoring life is difficult." [5]

We can find ways to satisfy our hunger without bogging our bodies and brains down into that slump. Our bodies have their own wisdom, created to signal us to want whatever they need. When we need water, we get a headache or become thirsty. Taking care of our bodies can be as easy as responding to those felt needs with healthy choices. For example, we can avoid high-sugar drinks or those with significant amounts of caffeine or alcohol if we prepare ahead to have healthy alternatives handy. Your experience may have already shown you that both the brain and body spiral down a dismal path after excesses of those choices.

Drink to Your Brain Health

We know we need to get enough water through drinking or the food we eat. Other drinks also pack a nutritional punch for the brain, particularly green tea.

Green tea has satisfied our ancestors' thirst and provided other benefits for centuries. But there's more, according to Massachusetts General Hospital's David Mischoulou, MD, PhD. He encourages regular drinking of green tea to reduce rates of certain cancer types and protect the green tea drinker from strokes and aging's effects on the brain. Researchers also credit improved memory and healthier levels of "bad" cholesterol to the tasty drink.

The secret to its benefits lies in powerful antioxidants found in plants called *polyphenols* which work, particularly in the brain, to limit the accumulation of damaging byproducts of metabolic processes. Free radicals are created when the body changes food into usable fuel. They are highly reactive molecules that can damage or destroy cells, and they are often associated with aging and disease. "A large percentage of the polyphenols contained in green tea have direct access to the brain, where they help protect neurons from free radicals and toxins, promote the generation of new brain cells, reduce the formation of toxic beta-amyloid plaque that is a hallmark of Alzheimer's disease (AD), slow brain aging, and perform other important functions."[6]

Green tea—fresh, not bottled—is my favorite source of caffeine. It's iced in the summer. In cooler weather it's hot with honey and lemon. And it's also good for the brain!

Here are some additional brain-healthy drinks:[7]

- Beet juice has been shown to lower blood pressure and reduce the risk of stroke. It also helps increase blood flow to the white matter of the frontal lobes of the brain. Health food stores often carry the juice, or you can make your own with a juicer at home.
- Carrot juice is a good source of *luteolin*, which reduces levels of inflammation in the brain. Tests on mice showed better memory in people whose diet was rich in luteolin.
- Acai juice from the purple South American fruit has a powerful antioxidant to help neutralize high levels of protein toxins. This antioxidant, rich with *Anthocyanins,* has been shown to prevent brain aging.
- Red wine—one four-ounce glass per day or less—has an antioxidant that can boost our brain's performance and reduce our risk of dementia. The antioxidant is *resveratrol,* and it boosts brain cell survival, helps prevent cell injury, eliminates cell-damaging free radicals and improves the blood supply to cells.[8]

"Eat the Rainbow" is solid advice for both drinks and foods. Choosing foods with vibrant, deep colors brings our bodies antioxidants and other nutrients. Dark blueberries, blackberries, cranberries, cherries, stone fruits, pomegranates, beets, and orange and yellow vegetables prevent aging and promote overall health.

Healthy Fats and Oils

Not too many years ago, we were told to stay away from fats and oils that were thought to cause heart disease. Now research has shown that healthy fats such as omega-3s from fish, nuts, seeds, olives, extra-virgin olive oil, and coconut butter are good for us. They reduce diabetes, heart disease, cancer, and dementia. They lower cholesterol and triglycerides, and are powerful anti-inflammatory compounds.[9]

Each of these sources can increase the health benefits as well as the taste and texture of our food.

Two to three servings (three to four ounces each) of cold-water fish are recommended, along with other omega-3–rich foods to give the brain and body what it needs. Dr. Olivia Okereke, MD, MS, a physician at Massachusetts General Hospital's Gerontology Research Unit, explains why we need omega-3s in our diet: "Omega-3 fatty acids, which are highly concentrated in the brain, must be obtained through the diet or supplements since they cannot be manufactured in sufficient amounts by the body. Omega-3s are thought to improve immune function, suppress inflammation, stabilize the cell membranes of neurons, reduce the danger of clot formation, and lower risk of stroke . . ."[10] Dr. Okereke also points out that some dietary studies suggest a diet rich in the fatty acids may also protect memory.[11]

"If your choice is omega-3-rich cold water fish, some of the best sources among common fish are: salmon (4 oz. provides 1,200–2400 mg), anchovies (4 oz. provides 2,300–2,400 mg), Bluefin tuna (4 oz. provides 1,700 mg), and sardines (4 oz. provides 1,000–1,100 mg)."[12]

If meat doesn't work for your body, plant sources which contain Alpha-linolenic acid (ALA) can provide omega-3 fatty acid the body can use. Dr. Joel Fuhrman, M.D., recommends "consuming a tablespoon of ground flaxseeds daily, or some walnuts to make ensure adequate omega-3 fat intake."[13] Other plant sources include: mustard seeds, tofu, nuts such as pecans and walnuts, walnut oil, canola oil, lean meat from grass-fed animals, and dark-green vegetables such as broccoli, spinach, kale, collard greens, cabbage, Brussels sprouts, and parsley. Consuming any of these will provide the healthy fat our brain and body need to protect and lubricate brain connections. Lubrication—sounds like the auto shop! Actually, our God-created bodies deserve at least the amount of attention that we give our cars.

An Oil Change May Be What Your Body Needs!

We've known for years that saturated fats can lead to problems. Both extra virgin olive oil and coconut are good sources of healthy fat and have become popular recently with health-minded cooks. Avocados are another great source of healthy fat with extra benefits for the body.

The Daniel Plan recommends that we "Change Our Oil." Stock your pantry with the following unrefined oils that are good for your body and your brain: [14]

- Extra-virgin olive oil (EVOO): for low-temperature cooking
- Extra-virgin coconut oil: cold pressed or unrefined for cooking at medium temperatures
- Grape seed oil: for cooking at higher temperatures
- 100 percent avocado oil: for cooking, less of this oil goes further than EVOO
- Flavored EVOO oils: lemon, garlic, etc., to add some variety to your cooking

It's interesting the way walnuts resemble the brain, as do other plant products that look like the parts of the body they support nutritionally. The shell and skull protect their precious cargo, the two halves mimic the hemispheres. Of course the rolling surface of the nut's meat completes the analogy. Nuts are another plant source of healthy fats for our brains and bodies. That list includes walnuts, almonds, and many others. They add flavor and texture as well as a nutritional boost with their plant-based protein.

Protein and the Brain

Why does our brain need protein? Good question! Neurotransmitters are built from the protein in the food you eat. These are important chemicals created and released from the end of a brain cell into the synapse or space between that one and the next one in line. These brain chemicals either speed up or slow down the impulse as it moves to the receptor of the next cell. "Most neurotransmitters are made from amino acids obtained from the protein in food you consume. Neurotransmitters are the brain chemicals that motivate or sedate, focus or frustrate. Their complex interaction is what shifts your mood and changes your mind. Neurotransmitters wag the tail of tadpoles and wage the tale of humanity." [15]

So, we need to find a protein source that works for our own body. Nutritionists recommend that we get protein at every meal to balance our blood sugar and experience fewer cravings. It can come from beef, pork, chicken, fish, yogurt, eggs, milk, cottage cheeses, or vegan options.

Beans of all kinds are efficient sources of protein for those whose systems struggle with meats. According to WebMD, "More than just a meat substitute, beans are so nutritious that the latest dietary guidelines recommend tripling their current intake from one to three cups per week . . . . Beans are comparable to meat when it comes to calories, says Dawn Jackson Blatner, RD, a registered dietitian at Northwestern Memorial Hospital's Wellness Institute in Chicago and a spokeswoman for the American Dietetic Association. But beans really shine in terms of fiber and water content, two ingredients that make you feel fuller, faster. Adding beans to your diet helps cut calories without feeling deprived." [16]

Consider nuts as another option. They multitask nutritionally, adding taste and texture along with both healthy fats and a good source of protein. How's that for a win-win?

Whatever the protein choice, recent nutritional research has generated guidelines for our food choices. The Daniel Plan describes the "Perfect Plate":

- 25 percent protein
- 50 percent non-starchy veggies

- 25 percent healthy starch or whole grains
- Side of low glycemic fruit
- Water or herbal tea to drink[17]

Body knowledge is power. Dr. Daniel Amen's *Use Your Brain to Change Your Age* recommends that we know and respond to these important numbers regarding our health:[18]

1. Know your body-mass index (BMI). Being obese has been associated with less brain tissue and lower brain activity.
2. Get your five to ten fruits and veggies per day.
3. Get eight hours of sleep every night.
4. Check your blood pressure often and make sure it is under control.
5. If you smoke—quit.
6. I am not a fan of alcohol intake, because of what I see on brain scans. Don't overdo it.
7. Get a complete blood count. Low blood count can make you feel anxious and tired and affect your memory.
8. Get a general metabolic panel.
9. Get an HgA1c test. It shows your average blood sugar levels.
10. Check your 25-hydroxy vitamin D level. This is critical and easy to fix. Also check your folic acid and B_{12} levels. A deficiency in these vitamins can add to cognitive decline.
11. Know your thyroid levels. Low-thyroid hormone levels decreases overall brain activity.
12. Find out your C-reactive protein level, a measure of inflammation. Follow a low-inflammatory diet.
13. Find out your homocysteine levels.

As with all recommendations, your doctor's advice and your own experience should be the final judge. Paying attention to your own body's reaction to food choices will guide you to what works best for your own well-being.

Nutritional Hazards

Pesticides have been shown to change brain cells' behavior, increasing the risk of Parkinson's disease. "The fewer pesticides you're exposed to, the better," according to Chensbeng Lu of Harvard's School of Public Health.[19] Local produce from farmers markets have lower pesticide levels, and buying from them also supports local farmers. For year-round healthy eating, many families have chosen to go organic, despite the higher cost of the food. UCLA researchers have documented the link between pesticides and Parkinson's disease. They "found that pesticides change brain cells' behavior—thus upping the risk of the disease—at lower exposure levels than previously thought," according to Lu.

"Avoiding pesticides protects us from *endocrine disruptors*, which are chemicals that throw your body's hormones out of whack, potentially wreaking havoc on essential bodily functions. Endocrine disruptors show up in pesticides, plastics, and furniture containing flame retardants."[20]

Making careful nutritional decisions pays off in the long run, with more vibrant health and vitality. Some nutritionists recommend, "If it grows on a plant, enjoy it. If it comes from a plant, avoid it." So many of our diets consist mostly of food that comes wrapped in manufacturers' packaging with disguised ingredients and mystery names.

Sugar has been called one of "The White Menaces."[21] The American Heart Association believes our consumption of increasing amounts of all forms of sugar as one of the biggest threats to our health. In the 1800s, the average person consumed 5 pounds per year.[22] Today's average American consumes 22 to 30 teaspoons of sugar every day,[23] while hunter gatherers used to consume 22 teaspoons in a year![24]

To make matters more complicated, sugar comes in many forms, and often under aliases. Christiano Lima goes into detail with slides posted online listing "The 57 Names of Sugar: You Can Only Avoid It if You Know Where to Look." The short list includes high-fructose corn syrup, honey, brown rice syrup, brown sugar, cane sugar, caramel, bet sugar, agave nectar, corn sweetener, lactose, sucrose, and molasses.[25] Glucose is essential for healthy brain function, but the body makes its own from the food we eat. Dr. Rachel Johnson, Bickford Professor of Nutrition at the University of Vermont in Burlington and volunteer for the

American Heart Association, says, "What does matter is that most Americans are consuming way more sugars than we recommend."[26]

What's most important is tracking and limiting added sugars. We must also consider the naturally occurring sugars found in whole fruit or milk. "You can easily avoid the added sugar in canned fruits by looking for those packaged in their own juices instead of syrup. . . . Remember that moderate use is okay in the context of an overall healthy eating plan."[27]

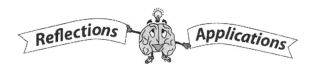

Reflection

Our bodies always try to communicate what they need. Have you ever gotten a headache when you forgot to drink enough water? Have you noticed any other warning signs?

Application

1. How do your mind and body let you know what they need? How do you respond?
2. What would you like to add to or drop from your nutritional habits? What is your plan for making that happen?
3. Try reducing the amount of added sugar you consume. Note how your body responds after a week or so.

1   Rick Warren, Daniel Amen, and Mark Hyman, *The Daniel Plan: 40 Days to a Healthier Life* (Zondervan, 2013), 26.
2   Horstman, *The Scientific American Day in the Life of Your Brain*, 72-73.
3   Ibid., 75.
4   Caroline Leaf, "The Power Of The Brain, Part 1," video, https://www.youtube.com/watch?v=U38eiCOy0Ow.
5   Warren, Amen, and Hyman, *The Daniel Plan*, 77.
6   Massachusetts General Hospital, *Mind, Mood & Memory*, June 2012, 4.
7   Massachusetts General Hospital, *Mind, Mood & Memory*, March 2011, 6.
8   Ibid.
9   Warren, Amen, and Hyman, *The Daniel Plan*, 95.

10   Massachusetts General Hospital, *Mind, Mood & Memory*, November 2012, 6.

11   Ibid.

12   Ibid.

13   Joel Fuhrman, *Eat to Live: The Amazing Nutrient-Rich Program for Fast and Sustained Weight Loss* (Little, Brown and Company, 2011), 133.

14   Warren, Amen, and Hyman, *The Daniel Plan*, 97.

15   The Franklin Institute, "Nourish: Proteins," Human Brain website, http://learn.fi.edu/learn/brain/proteins.html

16   Jenny Stamos Kovacs, "Beans: Protein-Rich Superfoods," WebMD, March 1, 2007, http://www.webmd.com/diet/features/beans-protein-rich-superfoods

17   Warren, Amen, and Hyman, *The Daniel Plan*, 79.

18   Daniel G. Amen, *Use Your Brain to Change Your Age* (Crown, 2012), 60–62.

19   "Health: News from Nature, Eat Organic for Brain Health," *Prevention*, May 2014, 22.

20   Ibid.

21   Warren, Amen, Hyman, *The Daniel Plan*, 107.

22   Tyler G. Graham and Drew Ramsey, M.D., *The Happiness Diet* (Rodale, 2011), 34.

23   American Heart Association, "By Any Other Name It's Still Sweetener," http://www.heart.org/HEARTORG/GettingHealthy/NutritionCenter/HealthyEating/By-Any-Other-Name-Its-Still-Sweetener_UCM_437368_Article.jsp#

24   Warren, Amen, Hyman, *The Daniel Plan*, 107.

25   Christiano Lima, "The 57 Names Of Sugar: You can only avoid it if you know where to look," *Prevention* website, http://www.prevention.com/food/healthy-eating-tips/57-names-sugar

26   American Heart Association, "By Any Other Name It's Still Sweetener."

27   Ibid.

6 MOVE IT!

Physical activity is cognitive candy.
—John Medina[1]

There's overwhelming evidence that exercise produces large cognitive gains and helps fight dementia.
—John J. Ratey[2]

So, now that we know how to get the right stuff into our bodies—managing calories in–calories out—what's next? I've always tried to burn more than I ate in a given day, and noticed changes in the scale when that didn't happen. Let's add another dimension that might spark renewed motivation for healthy choices. Move it for brain health! Somehow adding activity seems more appealing than counting calories and restricting food intake. We'll discover how exercise actually creates new brain cells and strengthens the connections between them.

Active Trumps Sedentary

Why stay active? Brain health is a compelling reason to include movement in our lifestyles. As our bodies grow older, we may feel less and less like moving. Aches and pains may coax us to do more sitting around. John Medina's *Brain Rules* cleared up many of my questions on this subject, so I'll share some of his interpretations with you.

He was intrigued at the cognitive differences among eighty-somethings when he compared an interview with Frank Lloyd Wright to another conversation he had with a man who lived in a nursing home. Their respective levels of physical and mental activity differed widely. Medina concluded that our level of activity is the most reliable predictor of successful aging. Our cardiovascular fitness, boosted by exercise, reduces our risk for heart attacks and stroke.[3]

But there's more! "Exercisers outperform couch potatoes in tests that measure long-term memory, reasoning, attention, and problem-solving skill. The same is true for fluid intelligence tasks, which test the ability to reason quickly, think abstractly, and improvise off previously learned material in order to solve a new problem."[4]

We may be "sitting ourselves to death." A study cited on CNN found the combination of sitting and snacking adds up to reduced life expectancy.[5] ABC News reported similar findings.[6]

It's Never Too Late!

The cool thing researchers discovered was that it's never too late to turn it around. In their experiments with elderly couch potatoes, results showed even four months of aerobic exercise could bring mental abilities "back online." And it doesn't take much—only thirty minutes, two or three times a week does the trick, and adding strength training ramps up the brain benefits.[7] Good news indeed!

So how does that work? Exercise gets the heart pumping faster, increasing blood flow to the brain. Sounds simple, but bumping up blood supply also gives the brain more of what it needs to work. It speeds mental processing and keeps your mind agile.

New Brain Cells!

Not only does exercise keep our brain cells strong, it even creates new ones! The five dollar word for that is *neurogenesis*. It happens in the hippocampus where most of our learning occurs. ". . . exercise increases blood volume in a region of the brain called the *dentate gyrus*. That's a big deal . . . . This blood flow increase, likely the result of new capillaries, allows more brain cells greater access to the blood's wait staff and hazmat team."[8] Love that analogy! It's amazing that the brain has a built-in system that works the same way a waiter delivers food to our table, and the hazmat team clears away the things that could cause serious damage—acting as the brain's busboy.

So how well does this crew do its job? We'll look at several studies from previous and current decades to see if they support the brain benefits of working out.

Research into Exercise and Your Strong Brain

Does exercise really make that much difference? Let's look at the research to find out. In the 1980s and 1990s, the MacArthur Foundation Study of Aging and America conducted a study that showed people who led a sedentary life experienced significantly more memory decline than did those who simply went for daily walks or climbed stairs at home.[9] More recent studies attributed their similar findings to exercise generating an important growth hormone, BDNF (Brain Derived Neurotropic Factor).

In a 2009 study by Arthur Kramer and his team, brain volume in executive function in the prefrontal cortex and hippocampus was found to increase in 165 adults who spent three hours per week for six months doing aerobic exercise, elevating the heart rate. These people also had better spatial memory.

Looking at long-term data, Kirk Erickson's 2010 study showed that these brain volume changes in 300 participants—average age 78—stuck around. This group simply walked during their study—nothing fancy. The researchers repeated their brain scans again three to four years later, and again at nine years. They found those who walked more blocks each time also developed still more brain volume in the prefrontal and temporal regions—where the hippocampus resides—as well as greater gray matter volume.

Working out bumps up the brain's production of its own fertilizer. Here's that hippocampus again—generating a growth factor that protects the brain from stress hormones. Medina shares Harvard psychiatrist John Ratey's reference to BDNF as the brain's "miracle-grow fertilizer". "It keeps [existing] neurons young and healthy, and makes them more ready to connect with one another. It also encourages neurogenesis—the creation of new cells." [10] During exercise, our hippocampus gets a boost of BDNF, making it easier for us to think. [11]

The most recent study in 2012 by researchers Denise Head, Tara Singh, and Julie Bugg compared brain volume in people who exercised regularly with those who didn't walk or work out. They discovered the hippocampus actually got smaller in the brains of people who did not exercise when compared with those who did. [12] Now, how's that for motivation to get up off the couch?

Brain Energy

We know we can survive only five minutes without oxygen, but why? Our brain runs on fuel converted from the food we eat. The blood delivers glucose, much like our personal wait staff. The brain is only about 2 percent of the body's weight, but it gobbles up 20 percent of the body's energy. [13] A real energy hog!

That part is easy to understand, but John Medina in *Brain Rules* explains the rest of the story. That energy comes in the form of glucose, a type of sugar created from the food we eat by stomach acid and the healthy bacteria in our intestines. All of the metabolic products the body needs then travel all over the body carried by the bloodstream. Frantic cells greet their supply with a feeding frenzy, tearing apart the molecular structure of the glucose to grab what they need. In the process of pulling this energy from the glucose—as in manufacturing—toxic waste results. "In the case of food, this waste consists of a nasty pile of excess electrons shredded from the atoms in the glucose molecules. Left alone, these electrons slam into other molecules within the cell, transforming them into some of the most toxic substances known to humankind. They are called free radicals." [14]

God thought of everything! He surrounded us with breathable oxygen— the brain's "wait staff and hazmat team" to obliterate the threat of free radicals, which would wreak havoc on our brain cells if left to their own devices. But our "hazmat" superhero oxygen swoops in with the blood to save the day—tackling the free radicals and sending them along with carbon dioxide to the lungs to be exhaled—if we get enough exercise. As we learned in chapter 5, brightly colored fresh fruits and vegetables also provide antioxidants, which attack those free radicals for us.

That's a lot of drama going on in our bodies—constantly. Ever wonder how we can feel exhausted after a day of sitting around? Without activity, our brains don't get to dump the toxicity and must simply deal with the internal threat without any help. That's a tough assignment! So get up and move! You'll feel much better.

Muscles and Memory

We know running and walking pump up the blood's fuel delivery system, carrying nutrients and fuel to the brain. But other systems are also waking up the body and stimulating the brain.

Every muscle has its own connection to the brain via spindle cells near the point where it attaches to the bone. The proprioceptive system, in communication with the vestibular system in our inner ear, lets the brain know all about our movement, balance, and our position in space.

Balance issues deserve our attention. Keeping our muscles and brain in sync can reduce the likelihood of falling and fractures. "To maintain your sense of balance, your brain coordinates incoming information from various sources in your body—your eyes, sensory nerves, and inner equilibrium center (vestibular system)—analyzes the information and signals your muscles to react in ways that keep you from toppling over." [15] Simply walking regularly on an even surface supports the communication between brain and muscles. Try t'ai chi! It's soothing and develops great balance. Physical therapists can provide specific instructions for other standing balance exercises. Add social benefits by trying them with a friend!

Movement triggers our senses and boosts learning and memory. Muscle engagement—even standing rather than sitting—jumpstarts the brain. Standing or treadmill workstations have become more popular for that reason. People have no trouble getting their recommended 10,000 steps in that way. We can take care of body, brain, and spirit by moving. How convenient! And simple!

And it's not only our large muscles. Exercising small muscles also stimulates the brain. Have you ever been annoyed with someone clicking a pen or tapping fingernails during a meeting? They may not realize they're doing it, but it's helping their brain process what's going on. Many people find learning easier when snacking or moving in some other way. Even chewing helps. Yep! There's a reason we like food during a tough mental workout. But to be safe, be prepared with healthy snacks—to avoid mindless eating.

Whatever your choices, make them with full awareness. Actively thinking about our eating or moving choices gives us better results than simply not thinking about it. Sitting passively in front of the television for hours has been linked with a decline in mental functioning.

Movement Breaks

A brain break during an intense work session can freshen attention and make us more productive when we return to the task. A study at the University of Illinois confirmed that "taking time to relax mind and body, even if it's only for a few minutes, can help you come back mentally and be present, alert, and focused on what you're doing." [16]

It could be a shift in attention or actual physical movement. When we move, stand, or sit with our arms and legs across the midline of the body, we are strengthening the connections between right and left hemispheres of the brain.

Long periods of sitting—like three to four hours in front of the television, at a desk, or in a plane—creates problems for the body as well as the brain. A study conducted at Indiana University researched the impact of sitting on cholesterol, waist circumference, blood pumping into the heart, and blood vessels' ability to expand from increased blood flow. "The researchers were able to demonstrate that during a three-hour period, the flow-mediated dilation, or the expansion of the arteries as a result of increased blood flow of the main artery in the legs was impaired by as much as 50 percent after just one hour. The study participants who walked for five minutes each hour of sitting saw their arterial function stay the same—it did not drop throughout the three-hour period." [17]

Researchers looked at the results of five studies that explored the effects of sitting and watching television on nearly 167,000 people. Then they turned to national data collected by the US Centers for Disease Control and Prevention on how much time Americans report sitting and watching TV. Based on all this data, the researchers calculated that limiting the time Americans spend sitting to three hours or less each day would increase the life expectancy of the US population by two years. Cutting down television watching to fewer than two hours each day would bump life expectancy up by another 1.4 years.[18]

So, we have several good reasons to get up and move for a body-refreshing five- minute movement break to keep the blood flowing.

Moving and Mood

When I'm feeling overwhelmed, a nature break helps. Going for a walk seems to clear my head, get me back into the present moment, and helps me pay attention to my body and whatever's happening around me. When I return to my writing, or whatever other task I'm focusing on, I notice new energy and inspiration.

Turns out there's a direct link between moving and our moods. Researchers have determined that exercise is helpful in treating depression—both immediately and over the long term. It encourages our synapses to release the biochemical that keep us healthy and happy.[19]

How comforting to know we can change our mood by moving. We don't need to be victims of our emotions, in the short term.

Depression and Anxiety

Sometimes sadness becomes extreme and hangs on for months. A professional will be able to distinguish between the "blues" and depression or anxiety. Exercise has been shown to be helpful with both because it helps regulate the body's chemicals that maintain our mental health.

"In one experiment on depression, rigorous exercise was substituted for antidepressant medication. Even when compared to medicated controls, the treatment outcomes were astonishingly successful . . . . The longer the person exercises, the greater the effect."[20] Of course, exercise is not a replacement for medical care, but it can help us prevent problems or become part of a treatment plan.

Long-Term Protection

We would all like to reduce the chances of mental problems in our futures. Medina notes that regular aerobic exercise cuts our lifetime risk for Alzheimer's by 60 percent, and reduces our likelihood of general dementia in half. Sounds like a pretty good return on your time and energy investment! [21]

Beyond that, Massachusetts General Hospital lays out the brain benefits one more time: "Research suggests that *exercise increases levels of growth factors* that promote the generation and survival of new cells in the brain; spurs the formation of new blood vessels; slows the progression of neurodegenerative disease; boosts mood; improves memory, decision-making, and other brain functions; and much more. Brain scans of older adults revealed that just ten minutes of moderate exercise produced changes in brain activation that were directly linked to improved scores on a test of mental ability." [22]

Your exercise plan can be whatever works and sounds like fun for you—something you'll enjoy so you'll actually want to do it. Of course, check with your doctor before beginning any exercise routine. He or she will be able to help you consider any personal issues that you need to accommodate in your plan.

Getting Started

However, *regular* exercise is the key. Our biggest obstacle may also be in our mind. Despite good intentions, habits are hard to change. These tips might make it easier to change our thinking and develop new habits that will last:

1. **Start small.**
   Find immediate, short-term goals that you know you will be able to accomplish. Examples: more energy, improved mood, less stress.
2. **Keep it simple.**
   Try walking or something else you can do easily without spending a lot of money.

3. **Make it fun.**

    Find something you enjoy. Don't set yourself up to fail by pushing yourself too hard.

4. **Get an exercise buddy or group.**

    If you make it a social activity, you can keep each other accountable and support each other through any struggles that crop up.

5. **Schedule wisely.**

    Try to find a time that you'll be able to keep. Avoid times that other responsibilities are likely to become obstacles.

6. **Commit.**

    Promise yourself that you'll stick with it for, say, three weeks. A habit takes twenty-one days to form. Just get there, even if you cut your workout to ten or fifteen minutes.

7. **Track your progress.**

    Create a workout calendar to note your accomplishments. When you look back at where you started, you'll be amazed!

8. **Celebrate success.**

    Once you've accomplished the initial small goals, bump them up, and celebrate measurable milestones. Examples: increased time walking, distance covered, working out more days this week.

9. **Defeat boredom with variety.**

    Mix it up! Add different activities like swimming and stretching or join a gym.

10. **Don't stop!**

    Keep it up even while you are on vacation or visiting the kids. Substitute another activity for your usual one if necessary. Just keep moving.

Workout Buddies

Of the ten tips listed, the most powerful one may be getting connected with a workout buddy or group. Laughter creates bonds, and increases the likelihood that we'll follow through on our plan. There is often no shortage of things to laugh about while working out with friends. We can find humor in our frustrations when we experience them together. Going it alone, we would likely have unrealistic expectations and be too hard on ourselves. When it gets tough, we may lose our resolve.

Our buddies would likely be less critical of our efforts than our internal "committee." The goal is to keep on keeping on, not to perform perfectly. Friends will nudge us to show up and give it our best shot.

For many years I tried working out on my own because my crazy schedule didn't match anyone else's. By the grace of God, I went to a different water aerobics class one day, and friends there invited me to join them for coffee. I made a permanent switch to work out with that group and, of course, join them for coffee and laughs afterwards.

This group of both women and men chose the name Water Babes so I could refer to them collectively for this project, and I thank them for their friendship and encouragement. On many Mondays, we number more than twenty for coffee, most or all of whom worked out together at the pool earlier. We celebrate birthdays, share joy, and support each other through challenges. On days when I don't really feel like working out, I go just to catch up with friends. Great motivation for all of us!

Exercising the Whole Body

The body benefits from variety. Different systems need different exercises to build them up. Mixing it up will also keep you from becoming bored with the same activities day in and day out. Exercises you can do at home are described on the National Institutes of Health website.[23] Seniors who prefer working out with friends enjoy the YMCA's Silver Sneakers program. Each of these areas deserve our attention and effort to keep the body and brain working at their best.

1. Endurance: get the heart pumping at a sustained rate.
2. Strength: working with weights builds both muscle and bone.
3. Balance: keeps us steady on our feet to prevent falls.
4. Flexibility: stretching keeps our muscles loose and able to move easily.

Exercise Options

Try some of the following to keep your body and brain working at their best:

- Walking
- Swimming
- Biking
- Tennis
- Yoga
- Pilates
- T'ai chi
- Circuit weight training
- Free weights
- Treadmill
- Elliptical Trainer
- Zumba
- Exercise aerobics class
- Water aerobics
- Curling
- Kubb
- Gardening
- House cleaning

Giving our brains and bodies what they need isn't as hard as we thought, and the benefits last a lifetime. When the brain and body are struggling, we see insurmountable challenges everywhere. But when both are happy, our spirit has a chance to soar. We'll look at the dimensions of our spirit in the next section.

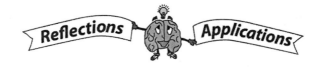

Reflection

What type of exercise works best for you? What obstacles threaten to keep you from being active? Can you deal with obstacles that get in the way?

Application

1. Choose a workout that you and a friend can enjoy together, encouraging each other to follow through on that important goal.

2. List ways to overcome each obstacle that you listed in the reflections.

3. Some people notice that working out affects mind, body, or spirit. Do you see any changes in your memory, your ability to think clearly, or your ability to relax?

---

1   John Medina, *Brain Rules: 12 Principles for Surviving and Thriving at Work, Home, and School* (Pear Press, 2014), 31.

2   John J. Ratey, Spark: The Revolutionary New Science of Exercise and the Brain (Little, Brown, 2008). As quoted by Dr. Joseph Mercola, "How Exercise Makes Your Brain Grow," http://fitness.mercola.com/sites/fitness/archive/2013/10/25/exercise-for-brain-health.aspx#_edn3.

3   Medina, *Brain Rules*, 22–23.

4   Ibid., 24.

5   Sarah Klein, "Too Much TV May Mean Earlier Death," CNN Health website, January 11, 2010.

6   Carrie Gann, "Sitting Ourselves to Death? Study Says Cutting Couch and TV Time Could Bump Up Life Expectancy," ABC News, July 9, 2012, http://abcnews.go.com/Health/cutting-sitting-tv-time-bump-life-expectancy-study/story?id=16743532.

7   Medina, *Brain Rules*, 24–25.

8   Ibid., 31.

9   Ibid., 87.

10 Ibid., 31.

11 Medina, *Brain Rules*, 31.

12 D. Head, T. Singh, and J. M. Bugg, "The Moderating Role of Exercise on Stress Related Effects on the Hippocampus and Memory in Later Adulthood," *Neuropsychology* 26 (March 2012): 133–143, January 30, 2012. As quoted

by Alvaro Fernandez and Elkhonon Goldberg with Pascale Michelou in *The SharpBrains Guide to Brain Fitness,* 2nd ed. (SharpBrains, 2013), 141.

13 Medina, Brain Rules, 28.

14 John Medina, Brain Rules: 12 Principles for Surviving and Thriving at Work, Home, and School (Pear Press, 2014), 28-29

15 "Fitness Counts: Balancing Act—Maintaining a Lifelong Skill," *Mayo Clinic Women's HealthSource*, monthly newsletter, June 2008, 7.

16 Ann Webster, Director of the Mind-Body Program for Successful Aging at Massachusetts General Hospital's Benson-Henry Institute for Mind-Body Medicine as quoted in *Mind, Mood & Memory*, October 2011, 4.

17 Saurabh S. Thosar, Indiana University "Taking Short Walking Breaks Found to Reverse Negative Effects of Prolonged Sitting," *Science Daily*, September 9, 2014, http://www.sciencedaily.com/releases/2014/09/140908083748.htm.

18 Gann, "Sitting Ourselves to Death?"

19 Medina, *Brain Rules*, 26.

20 Ibid., 26–27.

21 Ibid., 26.

22 "Working Up to Working Out," a *Neurobiological Aging* article quoted in *Mind, Mood & Memory*, newsletter of Massachusetts General Hospital, June 2012, 3.

23 National Institutes of Health, "Exercise: Exercises to Try," NIH SeniorHealth webpage, http://nihseniorhealth.gov/exerciseandphysicalactivityexercisestotry/enduranceexercises/01.html.

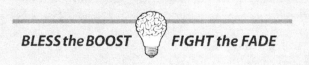

BLESS the BOOST   *FIGHT the FADE*

Bless the Boost and Fight the Fade: Your Body

Bless the Boost

- Problem solving: Experience pays off! Playing our cards right, we learn from our own mistakes and those of others. We've learned what doesn't work and some things that work better than others. That knowledge can be helpful when we run into snags.
- Body awareness: With practice, we are able to tune into the parts of our bodies where our stress shows up and give them the attention they need. Young parents are so busy with their growing children and have less available mental "space" to take care of themselves.
- Perseverance: Maturity often means we've trained our brains to stick with tough situations knowing they will get better over time. Aren't you glad we don't have to ride the feelings rollercoaster anymore? We can tell ourselves and others, "Don't quit! Your dream might be right around the corner."
- Reasoning: Gathering important facts and putting them together may seem to come easier with the years. We've learned to consider appropriate options, anticipate consequences, and make mindful choices.
- Willpower: We have a clear idea of what we'd like and often the resources to make it happen as long as it's within our control. Of course, some call this stubbornness, but it helps us follow through to our goals.

Fight the Fade

- Muscle tone: Our physical strength fades over time, especially in the muscles we don't use regularly. Keeping active even when we don't feel like it will maintain flexibility and health. Walking does the trick, as long as we know our limits and check with our doctors before starting an exercise program.

- Endurance: Can't keep going as long as you used to? Don't worry, you know you're not the only one. Stretching exercises and a light workout three times a week will help fight the fade.

- Sleep problems: "Sleep hygiene"—a bedtime routine—can help get your brain ready for its night crew. Progressive relaxation might make falling asleep easier. Reading rather than electronics and avoiding alcohol before bed should help you avoid a wide-awake bathroom break in the middle of the night.

- Balance: The brain and body's vestibular and proprioceptive systems work together to help us maintain our balance. With slower processing time as we get older, many people are at risk of falling. For safety at home, experts recommend clearing floors of loose rugs and clutter. Exercises to build balance, endurance, flexibility, and strength are available online at http://nihseniorhealth.gov/exerciseandphysicalactivityexercisestotry/balanceexercises/01.html.

- Hearing: Ear protection in noisy environments will help you preserve your hearing—for example, while mowing the lawn. Hearing aids can be a comfortable, invisible, and effective way to deal with hearing loss.

- Visual/spatial processing: Complex puzzles and geometric designs may become more difficult—quilters may have an edge on this one. Friends getting together to work on their sewing projects are fighting this particular fade, and their brains are benefitting from the social connections as well. A win-win!

Part III
THE SPIRIT

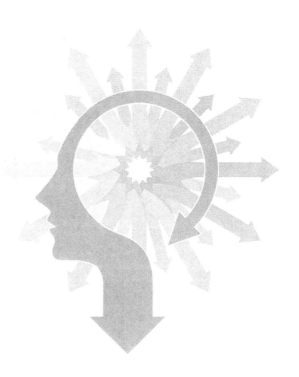

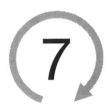

CONNECTING WITH GOD THROUGH PRAYER

Prayer immediately turns us into something greater than ourselves.
—**Cardinal Timothy Dolan**, Archbishop of New York[1]

Life to the full. This is the promise of the gospel. This is the pledge that Jesus makes to his disciples. Life to the full. This is the Christian word for fulfillment.
—**John Heagle**[2]

God speaks to us in many different ways, but we can only hear him when we are "tuned in." Wouldn't it be easier if he would give us written or spoken directions? We are accustomed to receiving information directly through our senses, but that doesn't fit his divine persona. He doesn't speak audibly, nor does he write his messages on a board for us to read. So, how do we tune into his voice?

He asks us to be still and know that he is God. That means turning off all other demands on our attention and focusing on him and the very personal message he has just for us.

Prayer: Speaking and Listening

Prayer is thought to be either speaking or listening to God. The spoken part could mean reciting memorized prayers, such as the Lord's Prayer and others which have been set forward as models for us. Or we call out to God, pouring our hearts out to him when we're overwhelmed and feeling lost, turning our pain and anguish over to him. We pause to thank him for our many blessings and carrying others' burdens as we lift their concerns as he asked us to do.

He wants nothing more than to spend time with us giving him our full attention, while either speaking or listening. Like any young girl, I knew what I wanted to "pray for," and wanted to jump right into giving him my "list." Patient, caring adults guided me to view prayer as indeed talking to God and as much more than asking for help. It's spending time in his presence throughout my entire day and checking in with him while making even small decisions. Take changing events for example. I began to see my interrupted or sidetracked plans as God's way of turning my attention back to him and his plan for my day. They became a highlighter prompting me to step back and ask for his guidance instead of resenting the changes.

Decades ago, our youth pastor taught us a four step "ACTS" pattern that I've adapted over the years, but still use to stay on track. The first three took some discipline for me to complete before getting to my personal requests. Somehow they open my heart and mind to connect with God more completely.

1. **Affirmation:** This means praising him for his character, irrevocable love, and constant presence, which have been constant throughout our lives. His presence, power, promises, and purpose lead us to our highest good if we choose to follow him. Spending dedicated time with him at the start of each day makes the rest of the day go more smoothly.
2. **Confession:** Every day I fall short and need to clear up whatever rift I've created in my connection with God before moving on.

3. **Thanksgiving:** Specifically noticing and being grateful for my many blessings opens my heart to receive his word for me.

4. **Supplication:** Asking for what I need and praying for others had to follow the other three steps, which prepared me to be open to his will.

A postcard from my aunt sits by my computer and reminds me to ASAP—"Always Say a Prayer" as I write. Historically, the acronym means "As Soon As Possible," and it brought urgency and panic. With this new meaning, I'm drawn into God's presence, the source for my message.

Let Me Count the Ways—From My Voice to His Heart

Prayer seems to come easily when we're struggling with something. In fact, that may be one of the benefits of challenging situations.

Researchers conducted a brain scan of a Presbyterian minister who prays every day to take a look at what happens in the brain during prayer.[3] To prepare for this fMRI , the technician inserts radioactive dye into a woman who is deep in prayer. The dye migrates to the parts of the brain being used during prayer. It tracks the activity of blood in the brain. Comparing the prayer scan to a baseline scan, these areas show as "lighted up" with brighter colors—indicating increased blood flow.

Researchers concluded that when Judeo-Christian believers pray, the brain "lights up" while we talk to God in the same way as it does when we talk to another person in the flesh. The attention area of the brain in the prefrontal cortex, and in the language center of the brain shows increased activity—through blood flow—and brighter colors.[4] Because atheists can't imagine a God, their brains show none of that activity. Believing makes the difference in the way the brain responds.

We've been given many choices for ways to send our voices to God's heart. He hears them even when they don't come with words.

- Memorized prayers: Established religions offer prayers that we may have memorized and use when we don't know what to say but want to reach out to him. The Lord's Prayer has been called the perfect prayer, speaking to all of our needs.

- Gratitude: Thank You God! Gratitude changes the way our bodies' systems work together, as we'll discuss in chapter 8. When we begin noticing all that we've been given, the blessings seem endless.
- Intercession: We see so much suffering among family, friends, and across the world. God has called us to turn those concerns over to him and to trust that he is in control of all outcomes.
- Help!: When the pain leaves us speechless, we need only call out and he will hear the cry of our hearts. That's enough.

Some prayers don't need any words. Sometimes it's just best to cry out, then be still and listen.

Listening Prayer—Be Still and Know

God has called us to be in his presence, whether it be speaking or listening, or simply being silent. Sometimes the "speaking" part is the easier of the two. Simply choosing to listen to God may not seem to be working at first. Turning off our productive mind and turning on the receptive mind takes practice. Sometimes *lots* of practice.

It may help to bring our attention to our physical contact with the earth, the chair we are sitting on, and the floor beneath our feet. That action brings us back to the only place in time that we are able to connect with God. Our breath is another gateway to connect with him. (See chapter 4.)

Try sitting in a comfortable chair and inviting God to speak to your heart. Begin with five minutes of stillness, and work up to longer periods each day. Focusing attention on breathing sometimes helps. It highlights the present moment—the only time period we can access his voice. Past and future don't work for connecting with him. (See chapter 4 for more breathing tips.) Inhale slowly to a count of five while saying "God" or "Peace." Hold the inhale for a moment before exhaling to another count of five saying "Love" or "Hope." Choose words that have the most personal meaning for you.

Some people find it easiest to "hear" God's voice through our senses… nature enjoying his gifts. The beauty of the sky and mountains, the bustling peace of the forest, the soothing feeling of water on our skin while in a stream, lake, or ocean, the feeling of sinking our feet into beach sand and watching his birds and animals going about their lives each inspire us to take a breath and wait on him.

His voice is a whisper that we easily miss when driven by endless tasks. We can hear it only in this present moment. Past regrets or thoughts of the future block our "receivers." Consciously setting everything else aside to listen to him tunes our mind into his message and guidance. He comes with a still, small voice that brings grace and peace. What a welcome change for our bodies and brains!

God communicates with us through people and situations in our lives—if we tune into those messages. Maybe the theme of forgiveness keeps grabbing our attention as in the case of Phil, as described by Fr. Albert Haase.

> For over a month, in all his devotional and spiritual reading, Phil kept seeing the word forgiveness. At first he thought it was a strange coincidence that this word kept appearing seemingly out of nowhere, in different books he was reading and then even one Sunday when his pastor preached on forgiving and moving on. As the days went by, and he reflected on his life, Phil realized that he needed to mend fences with his good friend whom he hadn't talk to after an unfortunate misunderstanding eight months earlier. He began to believe the constantly emerging theme of forgiveness was God's invitation to make a phone call. In picking up the phone and dialing his friend's number, Phil was selflessly responding to God's call in the sacred moment. And without knowing it, Phil was coming one step closer to overcoming the ego and developing the habit of self-emptying for the sake of others.[5]

Don't you wonder sometimes how many times and ways God tries to get our attention? Eventually, he breaks through and we get a flash of awareness. *Okay, message received.* Noticing is the important thing, no matter how long it takes. God is patient with us, even if we aren't as patient with him.

Living Prayer

Jesus wants us to pray "without ceasing." When I first heard that, it sounded impossible. How could we live our lives on our knees?

Billy Graham explained how this works. "The Bible says, 'Pray without ceasing.' If you have a special prayer period set aside during the day, your unconscious life will be saturated with prayer between those periods . . . . There should be stated periods in which you slip apart with God. For the overworked mother or one living under extremely busy circumstances, this may be impossible. But here is where 'pray without ceasing' comes in. We pray as we work. As we have said, we pray everywhere, any time." [6]

After many years of trying that concept out in my life, I believe he was talking about what I call "Living Prayer." My quiet time with him begins most days, but then I find myself inviting him along in everything I do through my day—writing, working out, shopping, cooking, cleaning, and spending time with friends. I've learned to listen for his personal messages within the context of everyday things that catch my attention. My take on his command for perpetual prayer is that he asks us to stay in touch with him, to run everything past his "litmus test."

It's a bit like my personal "spiritual malware" running behind all of my brain's programs. (PC users will relate.) I ask him to direct my path, to close doors that don't lead to his will, and lead me to those that follow the path he has chosen for me. I don't always appreciate the interruptions that make me change direction, but every time I come to understand the reasons for the roadblocks—in hindsight. Living prayer has led to this book, which has spent over ten years in God's "kiln." I'm offering back to God the gifts he has given and developed in me, leaving the outcome to him.

Knowing His Will—and Urgency

During my spiritual "recalculation" times, his answers seemed stuck in "No" or "Wait." I couldn't help wondering if I had misunderstood his messages. Trying to discern his will, I wondered if I had gotten sidetracked. Things that urgently grabbed for my attention seemed to pull me off course. Sheila Walsh's book *Get off Your Knees & Pray*, [7] came out in God's perfect timing. She offered three questions to help us know and recognize God's voice.

1. "Does anything in this situation go against the revealed Word of God?
2. Do I feel a great *urgency* and stress to do something right away? (italics mine) When I feel a compulsion to move quickly, I wait. God is a God of order and peace.
3. Do those whom I respect and trust sense God's presence in this situation too?[8]

These questions have helped me filter projects that seemed important—at least to someone else. Running them up the flagpole of his Word and that of my trusted advisors have helped me winnow the list and budget my time and energy wisely.

The year 1990 found me juggling family, work, and many projects that urgently demanded my attention. Stephen Covey's *Seven Habits of Highly Successful People* helped me sort out those urgent but not always important tasks from those that were important but took some time and planning to accomplish. Of Covey's four quadrants, the first one, *Urgent,* refers to crises, pressing problems, and deadline-driven projects. How hard is it to ignore the call of smart electronics—signaling emails, texts, friends' messages, or a ringing phone? It's a decision that takes discipline.

Covey explains:

Urgent matters . . . press on us; they insist on action. They're often popular with others . . . . And often they are pleasant, easy, and fun to do. But so often, they are unimportant!

Importance, on the other hand, has to do with results. If something is important, it contributes to your mission, your values, and your high priority goals. We react to urgent matters. Important matters that are not urgent require more initiative, more proactivity . . . if we don't have a clear idea of what is important, of the results we desire in our lives, we are easily diverted into responding to the urgent.[9]

The tyranny of the urgent can be oppressive, leading to inefficient multitasking and procrastination. Noticing my physical reactions to urgency has become a signpost telling me to slow down and figure out what's important—what is God's will for this situation? As described in more detail in chapter 4, I look to the pit of my stomach for my answer. If I feel pressure there, I know it's time to breathe, pray, and wait. Trusting God's timing has always worked out for the best. Tuning into my body also helps me stay in the present moment and on track with his plan for my life.

This Sacred Present Moment

According to Albert Haase, OFM, author of *This Sacred Moment: Becoming Holy Right Where You Are*, "God knocks on the door of this sacred moment as it unfolds before us. Unfortunately, we are often unaware of that knock until we look back and reflect on an experience in hindsight. God's knock can be as soft as an intuition or a gut feeling; it can be as loud as a need to which only we can respond. Sometimes that knock surprises even the most spiritually attuned among us." [10]

Perhaps we see or hear someone struggling and feel a nudge to be present with them, listening and bringing God's love to their situation. It could be a message that calls us to reach out to another person with compassion. Maybe it's forgiveness. For whatever he calls us to, he will also give us his grace to follow through. We become his hands and feet.

God calls us to be fully present in this sacred moment. Fr. Albert Haase says we must empty ourselves of ego, and replace the mirrors of our lives with windows to see Christ and the needs of others in our daily lives. Paying close attention to God's call will help us find the freedom to fully live. [11]

We must be still and listen to his voice, which leads us to the finer points of the listening part of prayer: meditation.

Meditation

From the outside, the meditative state is difficult to understand, which may lead many to be wary and resist learning more about it. Following our breath while sitting in stillness actually brings us in touch with the part of ourselves that may get lost in our urgent activity. Dr. Caroline Leaf in her book *Switch On Your Brain* explains the science behind what she calls "directed rest."

> When our brain enters the rest circuit, we don't actually rest; we move into a highly intelligent, self-reflective, directed state. And the more often we go there, the more we get in touch with the deep, spiritual part of who we are. I believe God has created this state to directly connect us to him and to develop and practice an awareness of his presence.[12]... {While in this state,} the brain is more active, growing more branches and integrating and linking thoughts, which translates as increased intelligence and wisdom and that wonderful feeling of peace.[13]

God designed the brain with a series of coordinated networks that are connected, work together, and impact each other. Leaf says that the nonconscious part of our minds is where most of the *mind-action* takes place.

Leaf refers to Richard J. Davidson's research to further explain. "What research shows is that when we go into a directed rest—a focused, introspective state—we enhance and increase the effectiveness of the activity in the nonconscious. Research shows that there is a greater increase in gamma waves, which are involved in attention, memory building, and learning, and there is more activity linked to positive emotions like happiness when we move into this directed rest state. PET scans and EEG recordings show portions of the brain bulk up that produce happiness and peace."[14]

Sometimes, grounding concepts in science can make them less threatening and easier to grasp. This principle is what led me to what I call brain coaching many years ago. One of my favorite descriptions of meditation comes from a twelve-step book: "In every quiet moment I can find to calm my mind and think through the day ahead of me, I am meditating. During these moments, by clearing my mind and asking my Higher Power to guide me, I find answers to my concerns. I don't always expect or enjoy the answers I get, but to turn away from them causes even greater turmoil."[15] We can trust his answers to eventually work out for the best for his followers.

God's Answers to Prayer

Billy Graham assures us, "Every prayer that you pray will be answered. Sometimes the answer will be 'Yes' and sometimes 'No' and sometimes 'Wait,' but nevertheless it will be answered."[16]

Remembering our reactions to situations—not the situations themselves—are the factors that create stress, we would be wise to "Let Go and Let God" *be* God. The creator of the universe is on duty, and we can relax into his care.

- Let go of expectations. He has an even better plan.
- Keep hope alive. He will get us through the very tough times—He's been there!
- Trust God's timing. It's always perfect—and we'll understand someday.

He who created us in his own image knows our needs. He will provide as long as we keep our focus on him. One of the best ways to stay connected is through an attitude of gratitude and trust—coming up in the next chapter.

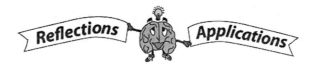

Reflection

Recall a situation during which you felt particularly close to God. What was going on in your life? Was it an easy or challenging time for you? How would you describe your feelings about this special connection with him? What was the outcome for you and for your faith?

Application

1. Each of us has a unique style for connecting with God. Which type of prayer "feeds" your soul?
2. Has God ever let you know that he wanted you to take some action? How did he get your attention? How did you respond?

3. How did you feel about the situation after following or not following his guidance?

---

1   Cardinal Timothy Dolan, *Guideposts,* September 2013.

2   Fr. John Heagle, *Life to the Full: Reflections on the Search for Christian Fulfillment* (Thomas More Press, 1976), 53.

3   Science Channel, "Your Brain on Prayer," *Through the Wormhole,* www. sciencechannel.com/tv-shows/through-the-wormhole/videos/your-brain-on-prayer.html).

4   Science Channel, "Your Brain on Prayer." Adapted from Jahnabi Barooah, "Study Shows How Prayer, Meditation Affect Brain Activity," *Huffington Post,* January 7, 2013.

5   Albert Haase, *This Sacred Moment: Becoming Holy Right Where You Are* (Intervarsity Press, 2010), 29.

6   Billy Graham, *Peace with God* (World Wide Publications, 1984), 170.

7   Sheila Walsh, *Get off Your Knees & Pray* (Thomas Nelson, 2008), 123.

8   Ibid.

9   Stephen Covey, *Seven Habits of Highly Effective People* (Simon & Schuster, 1989), 150–151.

10   Haase, *This Sacred Moment,* 63

11   Adapted from Albert Haase, *This Sacred Moment.*

12   Leaf, *Switch On Your Brain,* 82.

13   Ibid., 84.

14   Richard J. Davidson et al., "Alterations in Brain and Immune Function Produced by Mindfulness Meditation," *Psychosomatic Medicine* 65 (2003): 564-70 as cited by Caroline Leaf in *Switch on Your Brain,* 79–80.

15   Al-Anon Family Group Head Inc., *Courage to Change: One Day at a Time in Al-Anon II* (Al-Anon Family Groups, 1992), 173.

16   Graham, *Peace with God,* 169.

 # GRATITUDE AND TRUST

Hope is the thing with feathers
That perches in the soul
And sings the tune without the words
And never stops at all.
—Emily Dickinson

All I have seen teaches me to trust the creator for all I have not seen.
—Ralph Waldo Emerson

L ife happens. Everyone has a story. Lately, it seems that our friends and families have to face more struggles than ever before. Our prayer list gets longer and longer, and our supply of sympathy cards vanishes from the drawer. Challenges seem insurmountable. Our human experience is filled with struggles which can leave us asking "Why?" or "Why me?" How do we keep from seeing ourselves as a victim?

We've been told that the most stressful situation is the one in which we feel no control. Serious illness, long-term family discord, financial crises, and untold other issues send and keep our bodies in a dangerous "alert" mode. We know that stress wears down the body, brain, and spirit, leading to physical, mental, spiritual, and social problems. Can we find a way to throw the switch on our own tracks?

Remembering that our reactions to situations, not the situations themselves, are the factors that create stress, we would be wise to "Let Go and Let God" take care of us. Fundamentally, we need to trust God's timing and let go of expectations.

Gratitude

A switch to more positive living begins with our attention. Rather than reacting to difficult situations with worry or self-pity, we can purposely focus on something for which we can be thankful. God's blessings may be just outside our awareness.

We can start small, beginning by being thankful for something as ordinary as the snooze button. Who doesn't appreciate that extra few minutes of sleep? I am quite serious. Putting our senses on alert, we can begin noticing the colors, scents, soothing items in our homes, the blessings of music, and the presence of those we love.

Simply directing our attention to the positive things in our lives gives the brain a break from problem updates that we can't do anything about. The gratitude habit takes time and perseverance to develop, but our brain, body, spirit, and relationships will all benefit.

Let's look again at what happens when we are fearful. The amygdala—our internal homeland security device—sends a signal to release cortisol to protect us from the perceived threat. That's important when we're facing a saber-toothed tiger or physical danger. We need all the physical strength we can muster to protect ourselves. In short bursts, cortisol can ramp up our concentration and give us unbelievable strength. But when we live in a constant state of worry and anxiety, long-term cortisol baths wear down the body, brain, and spirit.

Shifting from fear to love restores the body and brain to peace. God is love. He can help us keep hope alive. He provides the antidote for fear in our lives. He will get us through even the very tough times. The best way I know to tap into his healing is gratitude.

Blessings Basket

During a difficult season in my life, a dear friend recommended that I keep a daily gratitude list. It began with writing, before climbing into bed at night, three to five blessings I wanted to recall from the day. Something very interesting happened. Knowing I would need to remember them at the end of the day, I found myself *looking* for things I would be able to write down. With my focus on positive experiences, I noticed fewer of the irritations and issues, and it seemed like the good things were increasing. Someone told me once that our energy follows our attention. With this exercise, my attention became uplifting. I felt stronger and better able to deal with the tough times.

My Blessings Basket still sits on my bedside table, with a different color of index cards for each month. I keep the cards together and am able to "mine" them when I want to write about experiences and memories that have become precious to me.

Dr. Bernie Siegel's *Love, Medicine, and Miracles* describes the benefits of positive focus.[1] Intense pain and suffering can make that seem impossible. Sometimes when I'm feeling down, I'm able to write a gratitude list, laugh out loud on purpose when nothing is funny, or give myself a sixteen-second smile. One of these exercises usually takes the edge off my discouragement, making it possible for me to begin climbing out of the pit.

God always provides exactly what I need at the perfect time. During my early rounds of chemotherapy, I followed a nudge to attend a weekend women's retreat. Thinking back, I know it was God's strength that made that possible. We prayed for each other and studied God's Word as applied to our lives. We talked about Ann Voskamp's book, *One Thousand Gifts*,[2] and the practice of making everything an experience of Thanksgiving or *Eucharisteo*. Voskamp offers many varying suggestions for noting blessings, including counting them up to one thousand on forms available through her website www.aholyexperience.com.

In an attitude of gratitude, my mind opens up to appreciate the present moment and everything it has to offer. My amygdala—internal security system—

is satisfied that nothing is going to harm me. My fear has said its prayers. Thanksgiving is a good place to live.

Being a planner, goal setter, and analyzer has served me well for most of my life. Studying personality development during my counseling training, I gained insight into the ego. A friend once explained that e-g-o could refer to "edging God out." I can recall investing a great deal of energy and effort into planning and trying to make things happen a certain way, according to my assessment of the situation. Guess what? It didn't work. Trying to make our own plans take shape can quickly obscure God's plan and purpose. Understanding life "backwards" made that clear to me.

Of course, planning is a good thing, but it's not enough. God is. As amazing as our three-pound brain is, I find mine to be useless unless tethered to its creator. Trust tempers the urgency of my plans and softens my focus on outcomes that once seemed so important. I've come to prefer leaning on God rather than on my own understanding—most of the time.

The Trust Chronicles

Let me tell you some stories that will illustrate how God taught me about trust.

Health

As I mentioned in chapter 4, my husband and I were forced to let go of our expectations when we were both diagnosed with cancer within a month of each other. We learned quickly that we are not in control of our lives. What a pair we were! Switching roles between caregiver and care receiver marked most of that year.

What a bleak winter! Long nights were even longer that year. Reading wasn't an option. I wasn't able to keep the storyline in my head from start to finish of even one page. PBS Nature videos will always take me back to those endless foggy hours.

But we were not alone. God provided everything we needed, and we learned to let go of things that used to seem important. During those months, we experienced God with skin on through many people who helped us get through tough times. My Bible Study Small Group and other special friends became the center of my life. They are friends in the truest sense of the word. They drove me to treatments when my husband just couldn't spend any additional time in the cancer clinic. They provided food, transportation, and company in a very special way.

Our daughters' families brought special cards the kids made and helped with seasonal chores that we were unable to do for ourselves. Time with grandchildren healed my spirit in very special ways. We will always be grateful for Skype visits and their wonderful, loving messages.

Diann, my cancer coach, answered my many personal questions and graciously listened with understanding when I needed to vent. She understood. She had been there. Another God-gift.

Prayers of friends and family brought a peace unlike anything I'd ever experienced. We had a physical sensation of being lighter as prayers lifted us up during those long days—and longer nights.

My first reaction after the panic was, "I guess God still thinks he can teach me something." As the song says, "We're all just one phone call from our knees." Learning to trust when our health failed was a journey we wouldn't have signed up for, but we did indeed learn some very important lessons. We both had been take-charge people. Suddenly, we were powerless. When we stopped striving, he was able to provide the best for us. In every moment, God was enough.

During the deep valleys of my husband's and my cancer experience, we actually found countless blessings, and my Blessings Basket cards hold the story seeds. I felt actual physical relief when I was able to shift my focus to his gifts. Watching that happen showed me how brain-body-spirit connections are so complete that a lift to the spirit also boosts the body.

Professional Development

We soon learned how "trust school" spilled over into other parts of our lives. Funny how our mental filters change during a difficult experience, and we begin to see all experiences a bit differently.

When I first tried to share my research to help other people, doors kept closing. Agonizing delays peppered my efforts. Eventually, I learned to trust him. God's timing is always perfect, which we'll all come to understand someday.

My writing journey took shape through school counseling, the perfect niche for me. Clear communication was essential when working with young children and their issues. I loved the interaction and synergy in classrooms and meetings during those twenty-five years. Children's spontaneity and energy kept my brain active and upbeat. The creative parents and staff at our school supported each other in programming and problem solving. We learned from each other while laughing and interacting during brain coaching presentations. I grew to love speaking to public and educational groups. People would ask me to put the information into book form, so I got serious about writing. Conferences and workshops prepared me to write for magazines and chapters for collaborative books. I worked diligently to learn the business and hone my skills.

I wrote daily, and when I wasn't able to, I truly felt something was missing. The business of writing involved endless tasks—setting goals, keeping logs and spreadsheets, pitching to editors and agents, submitting manuscripts and dealing with the "pre-acceptance" (rejection) letters. The timing wasn't right—yet. One editor's explanation, "No one is interested in the brain," showed me how important it was to find out their philosophy before we did any serious work together.

My mentor, Virelle Kidder, guided me through the Christian Writers Guild apprentice course, which took much longer than I had anticipated because of my chemotherapy. Virelle's encouragement and helpful comments kept me believing and trying through all the challenges.

But, even with all my striving, the words wouldn't come. I couldn't concentrate. When I stopped trying, truly letting go of the outcome, God chose to move this project ahead. His love had to shine through my work. My efforts fell flat unless he was the center. My focus needed to be on the message, not the management. On good writing days, my thoughts and words flowed smoothly. I tried to remember that feeling when the tough ones came again.

Someone reminded me that God doesn't call the equipped; rather, he equips the called. He will guide my work so it will accomplish his purposes. My job is to stay with the task, apply the experiences and training he has provided for me, and trust the outcome to him. Lesson learned, for now. But I always find another one just around the corner.

Papua New Guinea and Kenya

My Aunt Lois was my first spiritual mentor, teaching me to trust God's guidance beginning with Bible School songs. She and I still connect by telephone weekly since my mother passed. She and Uncle Chuck served as missionaries to the people of Papua New Guinea and Kenya many years ago. They have leaned hard on God through their entire life together. In her own words:

"Everyone was there with no pay—volunteer—unless they knew someone back home who would send some money. We didn't worry about anything because we had to trust God for everything.

We just trusted God because he sent us there. We knew he would take care of us, and he did.

One time sticks in my mind. I hadn't been aware of any tooth problems in the twenty-five years since I got a root canal, but suddenly it flared up while we were in Papua New Guinea. I was in terrible pain, with no idea how to deal with it. A retired oral surgeon 'happened' to come to New Guinea on his way home from Nepal. He looked at it and told me I had an infected root canal. He fixed it, and I haven't had any more problems with it in forty years. If he hadn't come, he said I would have been dead in three weeks. God is so faithful!" [3]

Aunt Lois's trusting spirit has shown me God's character and revealed the remarkable ways he loves those who are obedient to him. When I call her each week, her laughter and prayers give me peace and comfort. She has an infectious laugh! Knowing she's praying for me through my writing brings comfort and trust in the process.

Listening to the two of them tell their stories made me wonder how they could leave their comfortable home and conveniences. Taking their two very young children and living in primitive Africa in the 1960s was an enormous risk! But they knew they would be taken care of and lived one day at a time. This takes a special kind of couple, God's grace, and an advanced brand of trust. Hearing their stories inspired me to make the most of the gifts God has given to me. One of my favorites has been the opportunity to travel and gather experiences in different parts of the world. I later got a chance for my personal trust adventure to take shape—exhilaration out of my comfort zone.

Kauai Zip-Lining

When each new year comes, I typically choose a word as a backdrop for my year. This year it is "trust." A January zip-line trust adventure was the perfect way to kick off my "Trust Year." Zip-lining has been on my bucket list for a long time, but I was losing hope for the chance to try it. Who would expect an oncologist would get the ball rolling?

Never a smoker, my husband had been dealing with chronic lung cancer for the past three years. For the previous three months, his lungs had been growing stronger and clearer with each visit to the doctor, even without chemotherapy. Our Oncologist said, "No chemotherapy for you this time, so go ahead and plan another trip. They apparently agree with you!" We called the travel agent that same day.

Hawaii was a destination we had wanted to return to since visiting Oahu twenty-three years earlier with our daughter's Drake University basketball team. We set up a cruise around the islands.

We chose our excursions well in advance to avoid last minute lines on the ship. Zip-lining! I visualized myself gliding above the trees enjoying the breathtaking view. Sounded like a great workout for my "trust muscle." The doctor recommended no high altitude exercise for Bob, so he chose a ground tour of Waimea Canyon.

Our shuttle van—more like a troop truck—bounced up the switchbacks, dodged enormous potholes on partially paved partially gravel roads, through a pasture and up to the first run, at the highest point on the island.

Bundy, our tour director, introduced himself during our bumpy ride up the mountain. He said he considered us his entertainment. "I love the looks on your faces when I tell you my stories!" Not exactly what this skittish newbie needed to hear. I vaguely recall grinding my teeth a bit on the way up.

"Gearing up" was another adventure. Thankful we didn't have to figure all the straps and clips out on our own, We were motivated to pay close attention to their instructions. We looked at each other, figured out the gear, and climbed into our harnesses. Our bright red helmets were just big enough to protect our brains from contact with the cable on the runs.

Our hardy group of nine climbed the stairs to the cable and the platform for our first run. Bundy gave us his rote memorized training talk, but we listened very carefully! "Just keep walking until there's nothing under you. Then sit down and enjoy the ride." The gear felt surprisingly heavy at first, but I was thankful for every ounce when it became my lifeline. "Keep your knees high and hands off the cable! Only hold the strap, not the metal clip above it. Just relax into the harness. It will hold you," Bundy said. "Steer with your knuckles. Turn them in the direction you want to turn and smile!

"Feel the tension on the harness and work it like steering into a slide when driving on icy roads." That made sense. Good thing he had spent time in cold climates like us. "Go ahead and take pictures if you'd like. Put your camera strap around your wrist so you'll be ready." Yeah, right! My brain was busy reminding me that survival is most important. I am a photo fanatic, but . . .

Randy, our "catcher," demonstrated hitching his harness to the cable, walking down and off the walkway, then riding the cable to the landing platform where he slowed himself, stopped, and released his clamp. Bundy explained the process again and guided each of us down the ramp for our first run.

I hung back—the last one of the group to take that first run. Bundy hitched the heavy hook to the cable guide, I took three steps, grabbed the strap with both hands, took a deep breath, and the ground fell away. I still can't believe that I walked off the platform at 10,000 feet! I held on to the strap with both hands and tried to steer with everything I had in me. I didn't want to come into the landing platform backwards! Yep, that's exactly what happened.

Gentle muscle-bound Randy inspired trust and encouraged us to relax. My heart was in my throat when I came onto the platform backwards, but I soon learned he "had my back." No need to worry about the right approach. Randy would slow and stop us when we reached the ramp on the other side. His strength, compassion, and patience taught me trust—even at those heights. No horror stories—just brawn and smiles. Security is a good thing!

Letting go at those heights? Seriously? Yes, I was shaky, and grabbed the strap as if my life depended on it—well, it did. But my strap and harness would hold even when I let go. A young couple—obvious zip-lining veterans — showed me how to relax and enjoy the ride. Trust the harness. After several deep breaths, my thundering heart slowed down. I reminded the fearful child inside that my energy was better spent enjoying the view and the experience. Drink it in! Save it to remember later!

The first run was the shortest. They got longer, lower, and more fun when I remembered to exhale and relax into the ride. We had a great group — lots of laughter and encouragement. The young couple with us always made perfect landings; both youth and experience were with them. Margaret and Bill and I took photos of each other before launch and after landing—proof to ourselves and others that we actually did this! Our senior members, Jean and Walter, quickly picked up the steering strategy. Jean had surprised Walter by suggesting they zip-line on their trip. This experience obviously lighted up her brain!

Bundy generously offered to carry our jackets in his backpack as the day grew warmer. He took photos for us, and cheered us on as we launched. Just to make sure we made it to the other side on long runs, he gave us a push as we ran off the platform. When he first told us he would be doing that, I panicked. But apparently some people have stopped in the middle of the run, meaning Randy would have to shinny out to bring them back. That would have been even worse! For the first time in my life, I was thankful for every bit of heft on my body. I couldn't imagine being stranded in the middle of the run, suspended so high in the air waiting for a sweaty rescue.

A hundred shades of green, mountain peaks, ponds, and waterfalls lay below me, but I was too busy trying to steer and land feet first to notice them on that first run. Bundy told us later that we had been on the highest point on Hawaii's garden island of Kauai. I was zip-lining! Woo-hoo! Cancer who?

Interesting thing about traveling: We can sometimes share our most intimate stories with people we meet far away from home. John knew what to expect from this zip-line company, because he had taken the same runs a few years earlier with his daughter. While we waited for our truck, he trusted me with his touching and very personal story.

He and his daughter had planned to come together on this trip, but tragically, she passed a few months earlier. He showed me a small plastic bag with a short note he wrote and a lock of her hair. He dropped it as he passed over the middle of her favorite run. We shared tears and a prayer. What an honor to be trusted with that very personal story!

By the fourth run, I let go of one hand, breathed normally, and drank in the breathtaking view. Steering didn't matter anymore. Randy had my back every time I landed less than perfectly. What an amazing rush! Now to "hang loose" for the rest of my "Trust" year.

Kauai Backcountry Adventures had healthy trail mix for us after our zip-lining runs. They also planned time for a swim at a wonderful mountain stream. We enjoyed laughing together, remembering personal highlights and minor screwups while we learned "the ropes" of the runs. The bamboo grove brought back memories of my time in China some years ago. Margaret and Bill and I took photos of each other, which are now in *Around the World in Eight Days,* the digital photobook my husband made to help us remember our trip. We laughed and joked while we waited for our shuttle back to the ship. I would love to encounter my zip-lining friends again one day. Maybe they might read this book and we could reconnect that way!

Trust brought me to peace in Kauai and back home. I felt no more fear, just exhilaration at actually having been there and fulfilling my dream. Of course, nothing could capture the expansive experiences we had in the canyon, on the helicopter tour, or the peace of the beach. They are locked in our memories and will stay there as long as we bring them back to remember, through meditation, stories, and revisiting our photobook.

Gratitude and trust flourish in a brain bathed in love. Together they can banish fear. Love and fear cannot exist together, like darkness and light. Fear shuts down our ability to think and relate to others. Choosing gratitude can bring our minds back to peace.

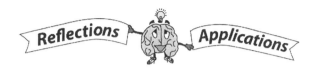

Reflection

1. Reflect on the influence of gratitude, trust, and love or fear on your well-being.

2. Recall a circumstance when you were unable to think clearly or remember what actually happened while you were fearful.

3. How does your body feel when you appreciate someone else or they express appreciation for something you've done for them?

Application

Create your own Blessings Basket or Gratitude List:

1. Find a decorative box or basket.

2. Get colored index cards, with at least 31 of each color, if you'd like the month's cards the same.

3. Scope out your blessings during the day. Your plan to write them down will help you keep your focus, and you'll notice more every day.

4. Record as many blessings as you can on the card. The trick is to notice new ones, trying to avoid repeating them. You might begin with three to five and increase from there.

5. During bleak days, reread some of the cards to re-experience your positive memory.

6. The website www.aHolyExperience.com has endless suggestions for you to choose from to creatively tailor your own Gratitude List.

---

1   Bernie Siegel, *Love, Medicine & Miracles* (Harper & Row, 1986), 147–156.
2   Ann Voskamp, *One Thousand Gifts*, 32–37.
3   Conversation with Lois Seldon, September 2012.

HUMOR DOES
A BODY GOOD

Each humor event you experience makes you grow a little bit . . .
the brain has expanded and taken on new connections.
—William Fry, MD[1]

You don't stop laughing because you grow old,
you grow old because you stop laughing.
—Fr. John Heagle[2]

Somehow, we can always trust a good belly laugh to help us enjoy our current situation. Humor actually gives the brain a good workout while boosting our spiritual and physical health. In this chapter, we will look at what happens when we laugh and why it's so healthy for our bodies and brains. "Appreciating a good joke involves a network of brain regions. Studies point to the prefrontal cortex as the front row audience . . . . Some studies show that the funnier the joke, the more active the prefrontal cortex becomes . . . .

Other studies show the amygdala (your emotional brain center) and the nucleus accumbens (pleasure center) and other parts of your reward circuit to be essential in appreciating humor."[3]

Sometimes true stories with a twist can catch us by surprise and get us laughing. My friend Diann got a call from a very responsible man vacationing in the Galapagos Islands. He had written her name in his calendar and wanted to let her know he wouldn't be able to keep their appointment. She didn't have anything on her calendar, so they brainstormed for a while. His wife remembered. "Oh, yes! You had signed up for that memory seminar!"

A Workout for the Brain

Wikipedia defines humor as "the tendency of particular cognitive experiences to provoke laughter and provide amusement."[4]

Finding something funny requires many parts of our brains to communicate and work together. It's a real workout for the brain. Here's a word map to show what happens in your brain in the fraction of a second it takes for you to belly laugh:

- First, the language center in the left brain takes in the words either from our eyes or ears—the occipital lobe or auditory cortex.
- The message zips across the corpus callosum to the right hemisphere side where social memories are stored.
- The hippocampus and amygdala check out the emotions and decide if you think it's funny or not. Personality makes a difference!
- The brain's pleasure center (nucleus accumbens) floods the brain with dopamine, and you feel good.
- Laughter begins in the brain stem when the dopamine shows up there.
- Endorphins flood the body.
- Your belly muscles—and others—respond, making you laugh.[5]

People find different things funny, depending on their personality. Researchers have shown that extroverts use the prefrontal cortex and orbiofrontal cortex. Introverts' brains light up the amygdala and front part of the temporal lobe when they laugh.[6] So the result is a bit different.

If you are good at remembering and telling jokes, consider it a gift and appreciate those who laugh. Their brains have had a good workout! If you're one who has trouble remembering or timing your jokes, don't take it personally. Keep trying with different people and see if it improves. Practicing laughter is a good thing.

Some also take a little longer than others to "get" the joke. Have you ever been in a group listening to a speaker when someone jumps ahead and laughs before the joke is finished and another person laughs long after the room quiets down? Everyone is different.

One morning, at our post-water aerobics coffee, one of the Water Babes shared a story that I'd like to pass on to you.

Eula and her family were seated in the front pew of the church waiting for her father's funeral to begin. She reached up to be sure the fancy hat she wore was situated just so. Her fingers slipped into a couple of the openings in the hat, and she was surprised that she couldn't feel her head. She gasped, and her sister Vera, sitting next to her, asked what was wrong. Eula told Vera the reason for her alarm, and Vera took a closer look. "Eula, you're wearing two hats!" she whispered, and both of them began to chuckle. The sisters sat right in front of their father's casket, struggling to stop laughing and settle down for the solemn occasion.

It turns out Eula's cloche hat had ended up nesting inside her dress hat in her closet. When she grabbed the big one, the little one came along for the ride. She was preoccupied with everything else going on and didn't check the mirror. These are the stories that get retold for generations.

Being able to laugh at yourself is sometimes easy, as in Eula's case. Sometimes it might be more difficult, depending on the source and intent of the comment. For instance, when humor becomes sarcasm, the target and others might hesitate to laugh. "Can't you take a joke?" that person may ask. Sarcasm can be thinly disguised hostility. Poking "fun" at a person or group often generates big laughs, but if they come at the expense of someone's well-being, that's where bullying takes over and the results are not healthy. Those who are sensitive to comments' hurtful nature are likely to refrain from laughter and perhaps change the subject to discourage further jabs. Keeping compassion in humor is likely to make us feel better than worse, the late Joan Rivers's barbs aside.

True Humor Heals

True humor, on the other hand, creates a bond, and connecting to each other is good for body and soul. It stimulates the release of neurotransmitters, dopamine, and endorphins, which make us feel great! Our brains actually connect in a special way when we experience humor with someone else. It's good for body and spirit.

Norman Cousins's best-selling book *Anatomy of an Illness: As Perceived by the Patient* inspires us to laugh for our health. Having been diagnosed with degenerative arthritis—a supposedly irreversible disease—he and his physician created a treatment plan during which Cousins took massive doses of Vitamin C and spent hours reading humor books, watching Three Stooges and Charlie Chaplin shows. It worked![7] Allen Klein shared Cousins' observation in his book, *The Healing Power of Humor*. "I made the joyous discovery," Cousins reported, "that ten minutes of genuine belly laughter had an anesthetic effect and would give me at least two hours of pain-free sleep."[8] Adding hours of laughter to any of our healing journeys seems an excellent choice. It certainly won't do any harm.

During "Max Your Mind with Humor" workshops, we laughed a lot while we identified our top go-to series reruns for our own version of Cousins's healing project. The groups collectively chose:

1. I Love Lucy
2. Carol Burnett
3. M.A.S.H
4. Art Linkletter

I pull out my set of twenty episodes of Carol Burnett on CD whenever I need a good laugh. It always works! From a health perspective, laughter works within our bodies to boost out health. The following is quoted from HelpGuide.org:

- Laughter relaxes the whole body. A good, hearty laugh relieves physical tension and stress, leaving your muscles relaxed for up to forty-five minutes after.
- Laughter boosts the immune system. Laughter decreases stress hormones and increases immune cells and infection-fighting antibodies, thus improving your resistance to disease.
- Laughter triggers the release of endorphins, the body's natural feel-good chemicals. Endorphins promote an overall sense of well-being and can even temporarily relieve pain.
- Laughter protects the heart. Laughter improves the function of blood vessels and increases blood flow, which can help protect you against a heart attack and other cardiovascular problems.[9]

Take a refreshing laughter break and notice how you feel afterwards. It might be fun to post humorous quotes and photos where you spend your time to get yourself started.

What's So Funny?

We respond to each of the elements of humor without thinking about them. That's part of its beauty. Disclaimer: What we are about to discuss may spoil the spontaneity of humor for you.

"Fish and house guests begin to stink after three days." Ben Franklin's quote illustrates different ways that humor works. Check out these ways below:

1. Odd pairings: Who would ever think of pairing spoiled fish with houseguests? The image catches us off guard and makes us laugh.
2. Familiar situations: I've been there! When someone describes a reaction we've had to a similar situation, we feel a connection with them that makes us laugh. "It's all about the door—not my age!" The event boundary story (from chapter 3) draws nods and laughter from everyone. Have you noticed that bills travel through the mail three times the speed of checks? Did I drive myself here? I don't remember any part of it!

3. Word budget: Less is more, or few words get more laughs than many. When people fill in the blanks for themselves, they are more likely to laugh than when someone explains too much. Ben Franklin's example used only eight words. Too many words spoil the joke. Sometimes too few words are just as funny: "Excuse my son for being. It was his father's fault."

4. Surprise: Timing is everything. The storyteller walks us down one path then suddenly shifts to something unexpected—and we laugh. Just when we think we have things figured out, there goes the "rug" out from under us. A short pause just before the punch line makes it stick.[10]

Visual Humor

Visual humor historically has been an effective tool for political purposes. It's a perfect example of all four elements: odd pairings, few words, surprise, and familiar current issues. The irony and satire in political cartoons lend themselves well to historical and academic studies. They economically communicate a great deal in a small amount of printed space.

We laugh when we recognize ourselves in cartoons and the comic section of the newspaper. They poke fun at everyday experiences and add a bit of levity to the often depressing task of keeping up with the news.

Visual arts—paintings, drawings, and sculptures—get their messages across with humor as well. Sculpture Tour Eau Claire has placed at least thirty original artworks on display throughout my city, replacing them with new ones every spring for the past three years. A vote is held, and one sculpture has been chosen from the tour each year and placed on permanent display at a site that fits the piece's subject. The bronze "Granny's Garden" stands near the Farmers Market pavilion with her apron gathered up and brimming with produce. Another Great Dane sculpture called "High Five" invites

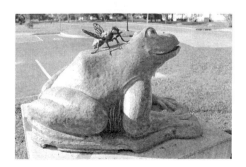

children and others at Phoenix Park to greet his upraised paw. One of my favorites is a frog and fly piece called "Blindsided." The fly perches behind the frog's eyes, just out of reach of its powerful tongue. Terrible tease! This one is also at a park and gets lots of activity.

Body Challenges

Sometimes we find it easier to laugh with others who are trying to do the same challenging task, as long as the stakes are low. During "Max Your Mind with Humor" presentations, audiences get into the nose/ear switch, typically triggering laughter. First we grasp our noses with one hand and cross the other hand over to grasp our earlobe. Then we switch hands, then switch again, this time more quickly. Adding eye contact and increasing the speed brings everyone into the experience, and laughter erupts, giving our entire body a good workout.

This exercise combines all four of the elements listed above. Eye contact creates familiarity and comfort, helping us know we're not the only ones struggling to accomplish the exercise—we're in this together. No words are involved at all, and people are surprised at the challenge. This exercise also builds and strengthens small muscles and brain connections with each repetition. Try it with a friend, for laughs of course.

"You Had to Be There."

Socially, laughter is even more contagious than yawning or sneezing. When the Water Babes get together, one person's shared experience launches an entirely new topic and guffaws all around. I'm afraid we can get quite noisy; but it's so much fun!

When several conversations are going on at the same time, the original group creates the humor together, but when others want them to repeat the story, the humor disappears. "You had to be there." It's actually very personal within the social context.

Laughter without Humor—Laughter Yoga

Turns out we can generate humor by participating in a Laughter Yoga group without actually needing to rely on our sense of humor. A friend told me,

"I feel as good after Laughter Yoga as I do after I have a good cry." She was amazed at the workout she got during a Laughter Yoga session. I had to check it out and went to Joyful Doc, Dr. Jodi Ritsch's class at The Center in Eau Claire. We began laughing artificially on cue, but quickly found ourselves in genuine belly laughs.

Jodi explains: "Laughter yoga usually starts with ten minutes of childlike playfulness exercises and laughing while making eye contact with others. When everyone is warmed up, and the joy chemistry has started, the laughter meditation—aka "free for all"—happens, which is three to five minutes of sustained laughing. Animal noises and gibberish are allowed, but no talking. This really amps up the chemistry. Then comes ten minutes of guided relaxation to feel all the great chemistry created." [11]

The "Guru of Giggling," Dr. Madan Kataria began Laughter Yoga in India in 1995. Now, over 8,000 Laughter Yoga clubs meet regularly in more than sixty-five countries. Using childlike playfulness and deep breathing, benefits of deep laughing are achieved while having fun. If you can laugh and breathe, you can do Laughter Yoga.

It begins with deep and full breathing—that's the yoga part. Make eye contact with others near you, then laugh out loud using your entire body. Fake it 'til you make it. Turns out, the brain and body can't tell the difference between a fake laugh and a real one. The physical actions soon trigger the same reactions as something we find funny. It's easiest to do in a social setting and with eye contact. Looking someone else in the eye makes a connection with both of your brainstems that gets both of you laughing together involuntarily. [12]

Laughter Yoga is a part of the Anderson Cancer Center's program for its patients. They produced a YouTube video that clearly demonstrates the fun and benefits of this amazing exercise. [13]

Five Benefits of Laughter Yoga

- Good mood and more laughter: Laughter Yoga helps to change your mood within minutes by releasing endorphins, one of several neurotransmitters or brain chemicals. You will remain cheerful and in a good mood throughout the day and will laugh more than you normally do.

- Healthy exercise to beat stress: Laughter Yoga is like an aerobic exercise (a cardio workout) which brings more oxygen to the body and brain, thereby making one feel more energetic and relaxed.
- Health benefits: Laughter Yoga reduces the stress and strengthens the immune system. You will not fall sick easily, and if you have some chronic health conditions, you will heal faster.
- Quality of life: Laughter is a positive energy that helps people to connect with other people quickly and improves relationships. If you laugh more, you will attract many friends.
- Positive attitude in challenging times: Everyone can laugh when life is good, but how does one laugh when faced with challenges? Laughter helps to create a positive mental state to deal with negative situations and negative people. It gives hope and optimism to cope with difficult times.[14]

Bumping Up the Laughter in Your Life

Why Laughter Yoga? "Just one session of hearty laughter is thought to activate certain blood glucose-regulating genes associated with the immune system for as long as four hours."[15]

Donna Peltier-Saxe, RN, Project Director of the Happy Heart Trial at Massachusetts General Hospital, says laughter is powerful medicine. "Researchers have discovered that laughter has many positive physical effects, including providing aerobic exercise, lowering blood pressure, expanding blood vessels, and increasing circulation, stabilizing heart rate, relaxing muscles, boosting the immune system, and reducing pain."[16]

Peltier-Saxe adds, "The mental effects of laughter are powerful too. A good laugh can raise levels of brain chemicals called endorphins that increase alertness, improve mood, promote a sense of wellbeing, and help reduce negative feelings such as stress, anger, anxiety, and depression among other effects. As few as five minutes of laughter a day can have a significant impact on our health."[17]

So how do we bump up our laughter factor in our lives? Peltier-Saxe offers some suggestions:

- Children are naturals—research shows they laugh up to 400 times a day. Spend time with them, watch them play, or better yet, join them!
- Gather a collection of cartoons, stories, and jokes and share them with friends. Humor is contagious.
- Check out the information at www.laughteryoga.org.[18]

For day brighteners, we would do well to see humor in our daily experiences. Laughter gives our spirits a boost, but we'll see that music can do even more for our brains and bodies.

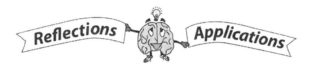

Reflection

Recall events when belly laughs made you breathless. How did you feel afterwards?

Application

1. Try Laughter Yoga!
2. Think of an incident when you felt better after a good laugh.
3. Come up with things to help you laugh as much as a child. How many laughs can you pack into one day? Can you make it to 400?
4. Thank someone who makes you laugh. Find a creative way to let them know they are supporting your health.

---

1   William Fry, MD, quoted by Pam VanKampen of Northern Area Agency on Aging, Eau Claire, Wisconsin in her presentation "Keep Laughing." Dr. Fry is also quoted (not these exact words) in Allen Klein's book, *The Healing Power of Humor: Techniques for Getting Through Loss, Setbacks, Upsets, Disappointments, Difficulties, Trials, Tribulations, and All That Not-So-Funny Stuff* (Tarcher/Putnam, 1989) 19.

2   John Heagle, lecture "Spirituality and the Human Journey" St. Bede's Priory, Eau Claire, Wisconsin, March 2, 2002

3   Hortsman, *The Scientific American Day in the Life of Your Brain*, glossy insert, 110–111.

4   Wikipedia, s.v. "Humor," http/en.wikipedia.org/wiki/Humor (positive psychology).

5   Pam VanKampen, "Keep Laughing," presentation for Chippewa Valley Learning in Retirement, Eau Claire, Wisconsin, April 26, 2013.

6   Horstman, *The Scientific American Day in the Life of Your Brain,* glossy insert, 110–111.

7   Norman Cousins, *Anatomy of an Illness* (Bantam-Doubleday-Dell, 1979), as quoted by Allen Klein, *The Healing Power of Humor,* 18.

8   Ibid., Cousins quoted in Klein, 18.

9   Melinda Smith and Jeanne Segal, "Laughter Is the Best Medicine: The Health Benefits of Humor and Laughter," www©Helpguide.org. All rights reserved. Helpguide.org is an ad-free nonprofit resource for supporting better mental health and lifestyle choices for adults and children.

10   This list was adapted from multiple sources and used in my presentation "Max Your Mind with Humor," given at University of Wisconsin-Eau Claire for Senior American's Day, March 19, 2013. Two sources I would like to note are Allen Klein, "Learn to Laugh Exercise" after each chapter in *The Healing Power of Humor,* (Tarcher/Putnam, 1989), and Ronald Berk, *Humor as an Instructional Defibrillator: Evidence Based Techniques in Teaching and Assessment* (Stylus, 2002) 6–7.

11   Adapted from Jodi Ritsch, MD, comments, Sept 2014.

12   Sandra Sunquist Stanton, "Max Your Mind with Humor," presentation, Chippewa Valley Learning in Retirement, Eau Claire, Wisconsin, February 25, 2014.

13   MD Anderson Cancer Center, Laughter Yoga video, https://www.youtube.com/watch?v=BrSABROitUE.

14   Laughter Yoga, official website of Dr. Madan Kataria, http://www.laughteryoga.org/english

15   Review published in *Life Sciences,* September 8, 2009, quoted in Donna Peltier-Saxe, "Laughter—A Powerful Medicine," *Mind, Mood & Memory*, Massachusetts General Hospital newsletter, February 2010, 3.

16   Peltier-Saxe, "Laughter—A Powerful Medicine," 3.

17   Ibid.

18   Ibid.

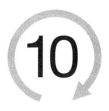

MUSIC MAKES
YOUR SPIRIT SING!

Music is a language that kindles the human spirit,
sharpens the mind, fuels the body, and fills the heart.
—Eric Jensen[1]

Grace, beauty, and music make cracks in the hard, impenetrable walls of
suffering, not always for long, maybe just for a moment or two. But in that
moment is the opening for all sorts of unexpected and inexplicable realities.
—Deforia Lane[2]

H ear that song? You can't help but move to the music! Can't get it out of
your mind? You're not alone! Music grabs the attention of the whole
brain and sends life through the entire body. It triggers emotions and
memories, and affects our general health all at the same time. It powerfully affects
our body, brain, spirit, *and* relationships, though it's included here in the Spirit

section because most people would characterize its effects as deep and unseen. Let's take a look at why music affects us so deeply.

Music and the Body

"Music modulates our body's stress response, thereby, strengthening our immune system and enhancing wellness."[3] Most people feel better when they listen to calming music. Eric Jensen suggests we look at "good vibrations" to explain how that happens. "It may be that the body emits normal vibrations when well, and aberrant vibrations when sick. When in a natural state of rest, the body vibrates at approximately six cycles per second . . . . This corresponds with the alpha brainwave state. Vibration rates might reflect not only our general health, but our emotional state as well . . . . One continuous feedback loop circulates information throughout the mind-body system. Every bone, muscle, organ, and gland in this system creates and absorbs sound radiation. Our bodies, in fact might be called 'bio-oscillators,' since at our very core we are composed of, and are emitting, continuous sound vibrations. Every function in the human body has a modifiable, but basic rhythmic pattern and vibratory rate that impacts our nerves through sound."[4]

The rhythmic element of music organizes the brain and enables people with tremors to initiate walking and modulate gait, people with autism to organize sensory information and respond without confusion, and people with dementia to respond meaningfully even after losing their ability to speak. Music brings the brain, heart, and other organs into coherence so they will be better able to work together.

The harmonic elements of music affect people emotionally due to variations in harmonic structure, tempo, and volume level.[5]

Stress hormones are reduced and immune boosters increase. Research shows that "music significantly lowers blood pressure in people who listen for thirty minutes a day to classical, Celtic, or raga (Indian) music."[6] "Moving with the music" may be a way back to wellness when we aren't feeling our best. It is indeed true that music produces "good vibrations."

Music and the Immune System

Music can also stimulate our bodies' chemicals to keep us healthy. It reduces our stress hormones and cortisol levels and boosts our immunity. Eric Jensen's book *Music with the Brain in Mind* cited a study that found that thirty minutes of music increased the body's supply of the antibody immunoglobulin A (IgA) in the blood, strengthening the body's immune system.[7] Music can decrease cortisone levels and increase interleukin-1, another immune booster.[8]

Creative surgical staffs have discovered that music can also support their patients' physical reactions during procedures. Another study focused on surgery patients "demonstrated the subjects exposed to music had lower cortisol levels during surgery than the non-music control group."[9] In the hands of healers, music is a tool with seemingly unlimited potential to help their work.

Not only does music impact the body, it also directly impacts the brain.

Music Changes the Brain

We know the ear takes in the sound and rhythm, but what happens to it next depends on the person who is listening. Personal knowledge and musical training change the brain and our ability to fully experience it.

"Studies of musicians dramatically confirm that the brain can revise its wiring to support musical activities . . . . Imaging has shown the volume of the auditory cortex [listening center] in some musicians to be 130 percent larger than the rest of us . . . . Musicians' brains dedicate more area toward motor control of the fingers used to play a specific instrument."[10]

Music activates and strengthens multiple memory systems. We use and develop at least four different memory pathways while experiencing music: Sight reading uses our semantic "what" memory; tapping to the beat uses reflexive (muscle) memory; encoding when and where we heard or played the music is episodic "where" memory; and learning to play an instrument involves procedural memory.[11] "Music gives us practice in paying attention, and uses our memory pathways as we focus on sounds, timing, rhythm, and patterns. What we pay attention to, we are most likely to remember. It strengthens both our retention and recall."[12]

Knowing the ways the brain responds to music helps encourage us to "apply daily and call the doctor in the morning."

Experiencing Music

We experience music in a number of ways: listening, singing, dancing, and actually making music. Listening always impacts my mental and physical state, either energizing, or calming. Singing along with the radio while driving my car reminds me of God's presence and blessings. Dancing has been a part of my husband's and my married life for these forty-eight years.

We respond to listening, singing, dancing, and making music in vastly different ways. Let's look at the way each of these affect the brain and body.

Listening

Music lifts our mood and keeps the thinking brain active even when stress and anxiety threaten to shut it down. The sympathetic (fight or flight) part of the autonomic nervous system revs up to protect us from threats. Listening to our favorite music can reverse that process, turning on the parasympathetic (rest and digest) system instead.

Lee Anna Rasar, MT-BC, explained,

Each generation of teens has a representative group who turn to different music from that of their parents, with this music more recently representing a style of music that is not appreciated by the older generation. This new music provides them with a culture of their own that is different from the past and may even serve the function of providing a way to manage stress. Very high energy music may be perceived as calming by them because they are used to busy and loud environmental influences and find comfort in what is familiar. In addition, their brains have recorded memories that associate the new musical style with friends and fun times.[13]

Perception is everything! Their music speaks to them and their experience.

Robert Zatorre, PhD, professor of neuroscience at the Montreal Neurological Institute and Hospital at McGill University, describes the dopamine release an individual experiences while they listen to favorite music as a musical rush. Imagine you're in line for coffee, and Pharrell Williams's "Happy" comes on the radio. The resulting cascade of mental activity it takes to process the music "touches on all the most advanced aspects of human cognition," says Dr. Zatorre. "First, the sound hits your ear, activating a series of structures from the cochlea (where vibrations are turned into electrical impulses) to the brain's cortex. When you recognize the tune—its name or where you last heard it—your auditory cortex is connecting with the regions that handle memory retrieval. Then, if you start tapping your foot, you've activated the motor cortex in a very particular way because you're tapping to the exact beat of the song. Finally, if 'Happy' has you feeling, well, happy, the song has turned on your brain's reward system—ancient, powerful circuitry triggered by essentials for survival like eating and sex." [14]

According to Lee Anna Rasar, "Music is holographic, meaning every association with the music is preserved—emotions, visual memory, smells, physiological body state (example: tension, relaxation)." [15]

Background music may also support learning for some children. Teachers I worked with reported improved productivity and behavior when they played classical music without lyrics during independent work time. The sixty beats per minute of baroque music nudges listeners closer to a healthy resting heartbeat. Less stress boosts mental capacity at any age. Students came to request music because it helps them focus.

Educators I worked with closely monitored students with special needs (ADD/ADHD/LD) for their individual reactions to the music. Some used personal headsets to play the children's chosen music. Others needed noise canceling to enable them to work without any distractions.

Singing

Each of us is able to listen to music, and we all have the basic equipment make music with our voices—with no reference to quality. Singing in the shower is a great stress reliever! Specifically, singing uses the left, right, back, and center of the brain "in concert."

To illustrate, let's look at the results of a study where PET (positron emission tomography) scans were used to determine where in the brain various musical elements were processed. Don't worry about remembering the names of the brain parts. The important thing is to know that music uses the whole brain, not just the right hemisphere as some believed in the past.

- Rhythm notes, language, and familiar songs showed processing in the Broca's area in the left hemisphere.
- Harmony activated the left side's fusiform gyrus.
- Timbre activated the right hemisphere.
- Pitch was processed in the left back of the brain.
- Melody activated both sides of the brain.
- Tonal processing is lateralized into the right temporal cortex.[16]

Singing in particular has the following benefits:

1. Boosts the immune system.
2. Releases endorphins that make you feel energized and uplifted.
3. Gives the lungs a workout.
4. Works abdominal, intercostal muscles and diaphragm, stimulates circulation.
5. Makes us breathe more deeply, take in more oxygen, improve aerobic capacity.[17]

Add to that list the emotions attached to each musical experience that makes it more memorable and helps us enjoy life. Who cares if we don't sound particularly musical? We can sing for our mind and body—not for applause. What fun!

Barbershop quartets combine amazing harmonies and lots of fun, which is obvious when they sing. Referring to those groups, Graham Welch of London's

Roehampton Institute says, "When you break into song, your chest expands and your back and shoulders straighten, thus improving your posture. Singing lifts moods and clears the 'blues' by taking your mind off the stresses of the day, as well as releasing pain-relieving endorphins. As you sing along, your circulation is improved, which in turn oxygenates the cells and boosts the body's immune system to ward off minor infections."[18]

Connecting the immune system to music may be a new concept for many. Another study at the University of Frankfurt in Germany revealed that immune system proteins and hormones were increased in the blood of people singing in a professional choir. The study concluded that people in the choir maintained strengthened immune systems a week later and that singing also improved their mood.[19]

Singing with a group has additional benefits. Another recent German study has shown that "active amateur group singing can lead to significant increases in the production of a protein considered as the first line of defense against respiratory infections and also leads to positive emotional changes. Given that every human being is, in principle, capable of developing sufficient vocal skills to participate in a chorale for a lifetime, active group singing may be a risk free, economic, easily accessible, and yet powerful, road to enhanced physiological and psychological well-being."[20]

Dancing

My husband and I danced the first day we met, and we still enjoy it forty-eight years later. My parents met rollerskating—dancing on roller skates—before Dad left for World War II.

To your brain, author Judith Horstman says dancing is a "neurochemical ballet, with the invisible choreography in your brain as intricate as that for any cast-of-hundreds Broadway showstopper . . . . Your brain has to figure out spatial awareness, balance, and timing."[21] The motor cortex orchestrates commands and signals to send to the spinal cord and on to the muscles to make them contract. Sensory receptors in the muscles send information about your position in space to help you keep your balance and follow the steps.[22] Then your brain takes in sensory information to gather touch and movement communication with your partner, which makes smooth, coordinated movement to the music possible.

Researchers Gammon M. Earhart and Madeleine E. Hackney of the Washington University School of Medicine in St. Louis found that tango classes led to better balance in people with Parkinson's disease and in the elderly. After twenty classes, they had better balance scores on the "Get Up and Go" test, which identified those at risk for falling.[23]

Couples who dance together communicate without words while following the music and each other. That forms a special connection that many come to treasure.

Playing Music

Playing the piano transported me into another world when I felt stressed or discouraged. I remember playing a particularly energetic piece while I felt frustrated—really getting into the crescendos and fortes. Listeners didn't need to know about the feelings that fueled my playing. And when playing isn't practical, background music supports whatever I'm doing—cleaning, reading, meditating, writing, or walking.

Music and Healing

On a personal level, our youngest daughter chose to become a music therapist, which meant that we could learn more about it while she was studying at the University of Wisconsin–Eau Claire. Lee Anna Rasar graciously provided specifics about music therapy for me during a recent interview. She cited the American Music Therapy Association's definition: "Music therapy is the clinical and evidence-based use of music interventions to accomplish individualized goals within a therapeutic relationship by a credentialed professional who has completed an approved music therapy program."[24]

My daughter's coursework closely followed my own search for details about neuroscience, with a bonus of unique ways of applying the information to help individuals of all ages. She learned to play many different instruments besides the piano and percussion, which she did so well before entering the university.

Harp Therapy

Harp music has a special appeal both for listeners and players. The harp's unique design lends itself very well to connecting brain and body. It is hand-carved and lacquer-finished hardwood. It differs from many other string instruments in that the layer directly plucks the strings with the fingers. There is no mechanism or bow that comes between the harp and the player's body. The motion of plucking the strings replays the grasping motion of a baby. The fingers also cross the midline of the body, serving to integrate the two sides of the player's brain. The neck of the harp rests on the harpist's right shoulder while playing. That happens to be very close to connecting right over the thymus gland—the center of the immune system. So, it's no surprise that playing the harp improves our overall health.

When our mother broke her hip, our family experienced the benefits of Harp Therapy during her hospitalization. She and we fully expected her to return to her home of nearly fifty years. We were devastated when she didn't bounce back from her surgery. We spent the rest of our time with her in hospitals and rehabilitation centers. Music had been central to her entire life—singing, dancing, and playing piano. She loved to tell stories about how she and our dad met and fell in love while rollerskating to favorite music before World War II.

While Mom lay in the hospital's ICU, we were surprised to hear harp music coming from just outside the entrance to her bay. We thanked God for sending the music therapy student to play for patients and especially for her choosing a spot so close to Mom so she could enjoy her favorite songs. The harp music brought a huge smile to her lips. My sister Pam and I stood on either side of Mom's bed and held her hands, singing along with the harpist using a songbook from the pastoral care department. Mom hummed along, even though she couldn't speak. That memory will always be precious to both of us.

Harp therapy had been one of my writing assignments for *Wisconsin West Magazine*. I was delighted to learn more about it and to meet Paula Smith, harp instructor at University of Wisconsin-Eau Claire and school psychologist for the Menomonie, Wisconsin School District. Her research with three- to five-year-old disabled children showed that "passive harp (listening to harp music) has calming effects, focusing children's attention and encouraging more positive social interactions. Active harp (playing a mini harp themselves) appears to support the children's language, social interaction, and fine motor development."[25] Harp therapy benefits all ages, and new applications crop up everywhere creative musicians want to support healing.

Paula told me about Ron Price of Elgin, Illinois, who experienced firsthand the healing powers of harp music. He had been a special education teacher with dreams of playing the French horn in a symphony orchestra. At the age of twenty-six, he learned he had a neuromuscular disease similar to Parkinson's. He and one of his students decided to learn to play the harp. The more he played, the better he felt. When he didn't play the harp for a few days, his family and friends noticed that he began walking with a limp and his speech was slurred. The word spread, and he now shares the harp experience with a group he founded called Healing Harps, a harp orchestra of individuals with and without disabilities, ranging in age from four to ninety-six, who gather to play together. Members of the group have become close friends, appreciating each other's company and helping when one of their members has a special need. Harp music brought these people together and allowed them to reach out to each other.

Music in the Political Arena

Who knows when people began using music to influence thought and political action? It was probably way before Civil War–era spirituals drew slaves together for their common cause. "Swing Low, Sweet Chariot" and many other energetic songs reminded slaves of their divine support and helped them deal with their challenges.

In our lifetimes, we can look at the civil rights movement. Singing "We Shall Overcome," Dr. Martin Luther King Jr. mobilized a generation to gather support for the disadvantaged. Remember "Abraham, Martin, and John?"

The Vietnam War polarized the nation, with music in the mix. Bob Dylan, Joan Baez, and many other performers sang for 500,000 people gathered at the Woodstock Music Festival of 1969, promoting the peace movement and protesting the military agenda. The "Ballad of the Green Beret" did its best to generate support for our fighting men and women defending freedom in the conflict.

M.A.S.H. began as a movie in 1970, and became a very popular television series from 1972 to 1983 satirizing the Korean War. The series' reruns remain popular with all ages.

The Singing Revolution from 1987 to 1991 may be the most dramatic example of music accomplishing political objectives. Through a nonviolent effort over the course of four years, 300,000 Estonians gathered and simply held hands and sang in unison their forbidden patriotic songs in defiance of the governing Soviet Union.

> On 11 September 1988, a massive song festival, called "Song of Estonia," was held at the Tallinn Song Festival Arena. This time nearly 300,000 people came together, more than a quarter of all Estonians . . . .
>
> On 16 November 1988, the legislative body of Estonia issued the Estonian Sovereignty Declaration. In 1990 Estonia had been the first Soviet republic to defy the Soviet army by offering alternative service to Estonian residents scheduled to be drafted. Most Estonians, however, simply began avoiding the draft.[26]

This nonviolent movement was the beginning of the end for the Soviet Union—triggered by song.

Bringing us up to the current music scene, a singing group called the *Capitol Steps* uses political satire to poke fun at both sides of the aisle. People of both blue and red persuasion find themselves laughing during their performances. At least for a short time, we can forget ourselves and laugh together—giving our brains a humor break through music.

Music and Relationships

Music also ramps up relationships when we hear the songs we sang together and danced to when our relationships were young. That might be one reason why oldies—now called classic hits—are so popular with baby boomers. Those songs were with us as we formed lifelong friendships. We smile and remember together a simpler time when we could understand the words and sing along. They had staying power from a wonderful combination of a great beat and memorable melodies. I find it interesting how today's kids are "discovering" and enjoying them as we did.

"They're playing our song!" Hearing those songs again all these years later can rekindle and deepen those relationships. Couples suddenly relive early memories in their relationship. Live performances of our special music sell out quickly to folks who want to immerse themselves in the mood of that time. While we can't turn back the clock, we can refresh our memories of those times by listening and dancing to the music we loved "back then."

Playing to music with grandchildren can also keep us young—or maybe just tired! Adding music to our time with them ramps up the fun factor. Children respond to music with unbridled enthusiasm. As a grandparent, I loved singing and dancing with our young grandchildren. We laughed constantly—a very healthy practice! It was a great way to build relationships and memories with my favorite people in the world, and laughing and moving together is a great workout!

Singing and dancing with little ones is one of my favorite activities. During Music and the Brain classes for toddlers and their parents and grandparents, we laugh, sing, and move together, enjoying rhythm and melodies and playing with scarves, parachutes, shaker eggs, rhythm sticks, and instruments. Families laugh together and leave a bit breathless but enjoy being together.

Music works its magic on our minds, bodies, and even our relationships. Take the time to play to music and enjoy it with the people you care about.

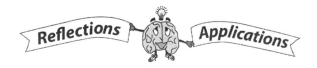

Reflection

How does music affect your mood, learning, and activity level?

Application

1. List your go-to recording artists for "oldies," workout, worship, and relaxation music.

2. What recording artists bring back favorite memories for you?

3. Remember learning the alphabet song? Are you able to recall anything else that you learned in a musical format?

1   Eric Jensen, *Music with the Brain in Mind* (Corwin Press, 2000), title page.
2   Deforia Lane, *Music as Medicine*, as quoted in "The Harp: Soothing the Mind and Body," *Wisconsin West,* June 2004, 13.
3   Jensen, *Music with the Brain in Mind,* 62.
4   Ibid., 63.
5   Interview with Lee Anna Rasar, MT-BC, WMTR, Neurologic Music Therapy, Fellow and Professor, lecture at University of Wisconsin-Eau Claire Spring Semester, 2014.
6   Horstman, *Scientific American Day in the Life of the Brain,* 127.
7   David C. McClelland, C. Alexander, and E. Marks, "The Need for Power, Stress, Immune Function and Illness Among Male Prisoners," *Journal of Abnormal Psychology* 10(1980): 93–102, as quoted in Eric Jensen, *Music with the Brain in Mind* (Corwin Press, 2000), 66.
8   D. Bartlett, D. Kaufman, and R. Smeltekop, "The Effects of Music Listening and Perceived Sensory Experiences on the Immune System as Measured by Interleukin–1 and Cortisol," *Journal of Music Therapy* 30(1993): 194–209, as quoted in Eric Jensen, *Music with the Brain in Mind,* 64.
9   J. Escher, U. Hohmann, L. Anthenien, E. Dayer, C. Bosshard, and R. Gaillard, "Music During Gastroscopy (German) Schweitz," *Med. Wohenschrift* 123(1993): 1354–1358 as cited in Jensen, *Music with the Brain in Mind,* 64.
10 Horstman, *The Scientific American Day in the Life of Your Brain,* 127.
11 Jensen, *Music with the Brain in Mind,* 70.
12 Ibid., 69.
13 Interview with Lee Anna Rasar.
14 Kimberly Hiss, "The Beautiful Life of Your Brain," *Reader's Digest,* 84.

15   Interview with Lee Anna Rasar.

16   Jensen, *Music with the Brain in Mind*, 12, 67.

17   Lee Anna Rasar, "Benefits of Singing," interview at University of Wisconsin-Eau Claire, 2014.

18   Graham Welch, Director for Advanced Music Education, Roehampton Institute, London, as quoted in Barbershop Harmony Society, "Health Benefits of Singing," March 25, 2010, http://www.barbershop.org/news-a-events-main/291-health-benefits-of-singing.html.

19   Adapted from University of Frankfurt study reported in *U.S. Behavioral Medicine*, cited in Barbershop Harmony Society, "Health Benefits of Singing," March 25, 2010, http://www.barbershop.org/news-a-events-main/291-health-benefits-of-singing.html.

20   Barbershop Harmony Society, "Health Benefits of Singing," http://www.barbershop.org/news-a-events-main/291-health-benefits-of-singing.html.

21   Horstman, *The Scientific American Day in the Life of Your Brain*, 128.

22   Ibid.

23   Ibid., 129.

24   American Music Therapy Association webpage, http://musictherapy.org/about/musictherapy/.

25   Sandra Stanton, "The Harp: Soothing the Mind and Body," *Wisconsin West*, June 2004, 12.

26   Wikipedia, s.v. "Singing Revolution," http://en.wikipedia.org/wiki/Singing_Revolution.

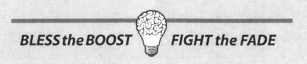

BLESS the BOOST   FIGHT the FADE

Bless the Boost and Fight the Fade: Your Spirit

Bless the Boost
- Trust: This one isn't automatic. Our trust gets stronger as we lean on God's gift of faith. We may have noticed that letting him run our show typically turned out better than when we tried to go it alone. Stepping forward in trust with those lessons behind us grows our trust "muscle." Life truly becomes more fulfilling when we lean on him.
- Gratitude: Over the years, God's grace has brought us countless blessings. When we stop to notice and appreciate his gifts, we can reflect on his presence through our lives. Doing so brings joy and peace to our brains and bodies.
- Focus: Retirement brings opportunities for sustained attention to activities of our choice. Our brain's ability to focus does not decline with age,[1] and with practice it may even improve. Find something that lights up your brain and go with it!
- Creativity: Many retirees discover and explore new ways of creative expression. Unlimited possibilities await us, and our creative drive either continues or gets stronger.

Fight the Fade
- Emotional resilience: Chronic stress can reduce our ability to bounce back from emotionally draining situations. The hippocampus, where feelings and memories are processed, actually gets smaller, giving us less available emotional equipment after dealing with long-term challenges. The antidote would be some combination of

exercise, meditation, spending time with positive friends, humor and laughter, and positive thinking.[2]

- Enthusiasm: Skepticism and cynicism appear more prevalent in the habits of older people. We may be less willing to embrace new experiences, concepts, and devices, opting instead for the familiar. Reversing that tendency takes open-mindedness and letting go of perfectionism. Enjoying the moment and letting fun surprise us will bring back joy and enthusiasm.

---

1   Nelson with Gilbert, *Achieving Optimal Memory,* 51.
2   Fernandez, Goldberg, with Michelon, *The SharpBrains Guide to Brain Fitness,* 141–143.

Part IV
RELATIONSHIPS

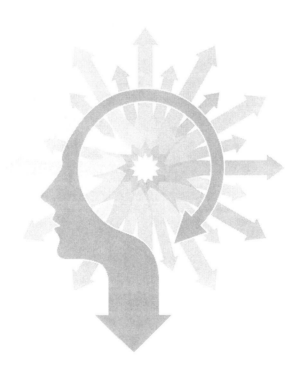

11

GENDER MATTERS

It's one thing to understand men and women in general.
It's another to understand the one you got stuck with.
—Mark Gungor[1]

So can all this help us with the people we know and love? In Part IV, we will look at our relationships with our spouses, friends, and families.

Since Adam and Eve, God intended for men and women to be together, to love and help each other. Decades ago, social science debated differences in male and female brains. Today anyone with a long-term relationship with someone of the opposite sex knows we don't process life the in the same ways. Living together in peace requires a certain amount of communication and understanding. When we take a closer look at differences in how our brains are wired, we wonder how that can be possible.

Developing Brain Creates Gender Differences

We will look first at the developing brain and get into adult issues later in the chapter. Remember hearing discussions about nature vs. nurture? At the turn of the millennium, this issue was hotly debated in public forums. Some believe male/female brain differences were caused by *nature*—i.e., babies were born different. Others insisted *nurture* was behind it—babies learned to think and act differently because of the expectations placed on them by their families and society.

Scientists at Cambridge University found a way to research the question. They gave newborn babies a choice to look at either a silent, live young woman's face or a quiet, simple moving mobile. "All 102 babies in the study were videotaped and their eye motions analyzed by researchers who didn't know the sex of the baby. The boy babies were much more interested in the mobile than in the young woman's face. The girl babies were more likely to look at the face. The differences were large: the boys were more than twice as likely to prefer the mobile." [2]

Researchers concluded that boys and girls brains are wired differently from birth—it's definitely nature. [3]

It Begins In Utero

How and when does that happen? Nan Brien, of the Wisconsin Council for Children and Families presented "It Begins in Utero" which provided biological background information to demonstrate that hormones and chromosomes, not society, create the differences between boys and girls before they are born! Between the third and sixth month, the fetus receives a surge of sex hormones, either testosterone for boys or estrogen for girls. "Boys get both X and Y chromosomes, whereas girls get XX chromosomes, which determine the child's gender." [4] The defining male and female chromosome combinations create the inborn differences in their brains. Neither is better or worse, they are just different—and they complement one another. God knew what he was doing when he created us male and female and asked us to help each other.

Males with their XY chromosomes are *systematic*. They are drawn to analyze, explore, and construct a system to explain how things work. If-then thinking creates patterns for them. Existing "in space" describes the way their minds and bodies work. Moving objects and activities are often their choices. For example, they like to create systems—like marble runs. Males actually need more space to move around in to be comfortable.[5] Hence, the "man cave" where they can be alone with their thoughts—and some mindless TV.

Females with XX chromosomes are *empathetic*, able to identify others' emotions. Their brains have more mirror neurons, special cells that help them to discern other people's emotions and respond appropriately. Language and relationships are female domains. Imagine an eighteen-month-old girl who focuses on her caregiver's emotions and may empathize, trying to comfort and soothe.[6] That may not happen with small boys—and maybe bigger ones.

Of course, this picture oversimplifies the situation for clarity. Many people, both male and female, come in the middle between systematic and empathetic.

Vision: Motion and Color

Taking X and Y to the next step, the structure of the retina makes gender differences happen. Who would have guessed that the eye would create gender differences? This will get a bit more scientific, but please hear me out. Biology tells us girls have XX chromosomes, twice the number of X chromosomes which process vision and color. Boys, by DNA definition, have XY chromosomes. Y chromosomes generate "cones" or motion detectors which girls lack. X chromosomes provide the color receptors in the retina called "rods." According to Leonard Sax, MD, PhD, in his book *Why Gender Matters: What Parents and Teachers Need to Know about the Emerging Science of Sex Differences*, XX and XY determine the rod and cone composition of the retina. "The retina is that part of the eye that converts light into a neurological signal. The retina is divided into layers. One layer contains the photoreceptors, the rods and the cones. Rods are sensitive to black and white. Rods are colorblind. Cones are sensitive to color."[7]

Simplified, we know the retina is made up of rods and cones. Rods are motion detectors. Cones distinguish color. Girls have twice as many cones, so they are able to tune into color more easily than boys who have only one X chromosome. With the motion processing Y chromosome sending more neurological motion messages to the brain, boys' brains actually develop a bigger motion processing "address." The brain adapts to what it has available.

These cell locations give females better peripheral vision while males get tunnel vision, which can create dangerous situations. Unfortunately, the guys are also emotionally drawn to risk. This is a stressful combination for the women who love them.

Nan Brien described an exercise in which she gave a blank sheet of white paper to boys and girls with a complete set of crayons and asked them to draw something. When some asked for more direction, she told them to draw something they did yesterday. They were to identify their picture by writing only boy or girl on the back.

When they seemed to be finished, she gathered the pictures and held them up for the group to see. Several elements showed up differing by gender.

1. Colors: Girls used ten or more bright colors, while boys chose at most six—variations of black, gray, blue.
2. Action: Boys drew verbs—things and people in motion. Girls drew nouns—still pictures.
3. Faces: Girls drew close-up whole faces looking at the viewer. Boys drew remote profiles looking to one side or the other.[8]

Researchers like to be able to replicate their studies—so I tried it with my students. Again, the boys used fewer and darker colors, drew either no people or only side views, and lots of movement showing risky situations. Girls made rainbows, flowers, and balloons with many bright colors, while showing full smiling faces. Interesting!

Of course, these observations are from unique but typical groups. We can't conclude that boys don't like color, and girls shy away from movement. Each of us is different and can enjoy the journey to our true selves. My brother's art is filled with yellows and oranges, and our eldest daughter is a successful engineer. Everyone's gifts are unique, and God has asked us asked us to explore and develop the ones we've been given. . Of course, generalizations always have exceptions. A mother told me about her surprise when her boy-girl twins' personalities reflected the opposite of researched gender principles. Maybe the exception truly proves the rule?

Dr. Sax described another classroom situation during which a boy drew a picture of a crashing rocket with only a black crayon. His teacher tried to coax him to add people and color to the picture according to principles she had learned during her bachelor's education training. Unfortunately, the look on the boy's face showed he got the message that the teacher wasn't satisfied with the drawing he was so proud to show her. Repeating that scenario may have led him to stop trying.[9] Understanding how children's brains work is very important for educators, parents, and grandparents.[10]

Vision isn't the only sensory system showing up differently between genders. Considering that every message into the brain comes with an emotional tag, our sense of hearing also brings variations in male and female language and empathy to our attention.

Hearing

Females' hearing is more sensitive and finely tuned than males', particularly in the conversational range, so they are better able to pick up tone differences in voices. Empathy follows for females, while the inflections may fly right past the males. Loud voices are particularly stressful for young girls. Women and girls may interpret communication as "yelling" when the men don't intend nor hear it that way. This might explain much of our miscommunication. It's important for us to notice body language and check for feelings to avoid escalating problems.

"Selective hearing" is tough to research, except through our own experience and interpretations. Have you noticed lapses in what the guys hear—or at least respond to?

Communication requires patience and understanding, as we'll discuss later in this chapter.

Language

When it comes to interpreting what we hear, males typically use their left brain, while females actually have areas dedicated to speech and language in both sides according to Nan Brien's research.[11] So, females have more "language dexterity." First, females have a bigger and more synapse dense corpus callosum between the hemispheres—a superhighway—between the right and left hemispheres. Pairing that with their double language processing areas, we can see how they are likely to be much more nimble using language.

Girl talk can jump all over the place with lots of emotion and description. Guys are more comfortable when we "cut to the chase." With practice, guys can learn to be patient and enjoy—or tolerate—women's "bird walking" conversations. Women can also learn to edit their emotion-laden monologues so the guys will be able to stick with them longer. It takes hard work, but is sure to improve communication and relationships.

Emotion

Speaking of emotion, it also shows up differently because of unique wiring. Females have more blood flow to the midbrain that processes feelings and saves memories. They also have more connections between the midbrain and the cortex or thinking brain and language centers. Together, these work to give females better ability to consider the context of a situation, understand their own and others' emotions, and express what they have experienced.

Studies cited by Nan Brien show that boys take up to seven hours longer to process situations that require complex emotive responses.[12] Remembering that their affinity for language is less well developed than females, we may need to expect less "talking it out" and expressing emotions than we find in relationships with other women. Guys may appreciate their women giving them a break and more time to process emotion-laden situations. The outcomes may turn out better for everyone.

So What Does That Mean for Us Grownups?

With that background in mind, let's look at our adult relationships. Over coffee, one friend might say, "I can't believe that my husband can just sit and not think about anything! How is that possible?" Or one of the men says, "How can she talk for hours on the phone to someone she doesn't even know very well?"

Our personal experience is our only point of reference for understanding each other. It's human nature to assume the other person sees things the same way we do. As we've seen from developing brain differences, that is clearly not the case.

Waffles and Spaghetti

Bill and Pam Farrel came up with a food analogy to explain gender differences in their book, *Men Are Like Waffles, Women Are Like Spaghetti: Understanding and Delighting in Your Differences.*

Men are like waffles: "Men process life in boxes. If you look down at a waffle, you see a collection of boxes separated by walls. The boxes are all separate from each other and make convenient holding places." [13]

Women are like spaghetti: "…Women process life more like a plate of pasta. If you look at a plate of spaghetti, you notice that there are lots of individual noodles that all touch one another. If you attempted to follow one noodle around the plate, you would intersect a lot of other noodles, and you might even switch to another noodle seamlessly . . ." [14]

Here's another tidbit about men's waffles: many of their boxes contain no words. Memories and feelings are there, but these men are unable to translate them into the words women need for communication.

Some of the boxes are completely empty. REALLY! That seems impossible to women, who have constant chatter running through their minds. When the women in their lives see them "just sitting there" it seems the perfect time to try to connect—which creates big-time stress for men. [15]

A Tale of Two Brains

Mark Gungor's *Tale of Two Brains* presents a different analogy that makes a similar point. He tackles the topic with humor, getting audiences laughing and understanding each other's mental processes. [16]

Paraphrasing his *Tale of Two Brains*:

A man's brain is a collection of boxes, each with a nice little cover. Each one holds just one part of his life—money, sports, kids, hobby, friends, relatives, etc. When has he has a job to do, he takes out that box, removes the cover, does whatever he needs to do, then slowly and carefully replaces the cover and puts the box back in its spot. He never opens more than one box at a time, and doesn't allow the boxes to touch each other.

A woman's brain, on the other hand, is a "jumble of wires connecting everything to everything else." Doing laundry reminds her of her mother, and she remembers she needs to buy her a gift, which brings back the warning that she needs to balance the checkbook, which connects somehow to social media, etc., etc. Each of these things is also weighted by either positive or negative feelings.

The part of his description that gets the most knowing nods is the "Nothing Box." Every man has as a box in his collection called a "Nothing Box" which holds—you guessed it—absolutely nothing. Our generalized man is perfectly content to spend endless time there, and resents being prodded to put it away, especially to talk about emotional situations.

Women, on the other hand, connect everything to emotions. They may interpret simple, benign interactions as revealing judgments. Then they are off to the races. "Why did my friend say that? Is she angry about something I did? How should I apologize?"[17]

Gungor goes on to point out that women's brains look for ways to "give" to each other—their friends, spouses, family, people in need. Men, on the other hand, love to insult each other. And their brains love to "take." He says women enter relationships believing they will be taken care of—an "over-romanticized" view of what things will look like down the road.

Women want to love unconditionally, but Gungor explains, "Unconditional love demands conditions. The stronger the relationship, the stronger the conditions."[18] He says females need to be empowered and learn to "take." Men, of course, enjoy "taking," but can be encouraged to "give" if their women actually tell them what they need and want rather than assuming they can read the unspoken body language.

Women might try Gungor's following four steps to improve communication and results:

1. Put it into words. Don't assume that he "sees" or "knows" what you want. Ask him more than once. "Men are takers, they don't *wanna* do it!"
2. Ask him kindly. Embarrassing or criticizing a guy only makes him more resistant.
3. Appreciate the things he does, even if they are expected. Positive reinforcement goes a long way.
4. Barter with him. "Do this and you can do that."[19]

Getting couples to laugh together opens the door to brand new understanding and acceptance. Gender brain differences in communication and understanding won't be a walk in the park, although that might help get things started.

To make things still more challenging, these generalizations may not exactly fit specific people—like the one you're with. Women's reactions are anything but predictable, and every man has his own way of responding to any given situation.

Communicating with Love Languages

This brings us to the need for discovering the unique ways our life partner prefers to receive our messages. Gary Chapman's *The Five Love Languages* details five very different ways men and women send and receive loving communication. We won't give away the details, but we encourage couples to study each other's style together over time. He calls each particular way of receiving love that person's *love language.*

1. Words of Affirmation
2. Quality Time
3. Receiving Gifts
4. Acts of Service
5. Physical Touch[20]

Identifying your spouse's love language may sound simple, but it takes patience, communication, and hard work. Chapman offers a clue for those trying to figure it out. We typically begin by reaching out to our loved one using the love language we are most comfortable receiving. Brain coaching tells us that the brain always goes back to familiar connections, so noticing how your spouse shows his or her love might be a good place to start understanding how they want to receive your messages of love.

"Lulabelle's" Laundry

"Why can't you just sit down and relax? You're so busy all the time!" The plea comes from friends' spouses who simply can't understand why women can't relax like men. It seems to go back to vision. Women's peripheral vision is *very* well developed, so we can see every little thing that's out of place in our homes. Together, those nagging visuals become an annoying to-do list that creates its own stress in their tired brains.

Personal example: I get urgent assignments every time I walk into a room. Everything that's out of place calls out to me like a toddler impatient for my attention. "Go through the mail on the counter! That jacket is still on the back of the chair! Hang it up! The newspapers need to go into recycling!" Then my foot gets stuck to the floor, and I realize someone had spilled something. "I need to clean that up! Get going on fixing supper!" So we fall behind before we get started.

To save time, instead of running something downstairs I might put it next to the railing making a mental note to bring it along the next time I go down the stairs. Then my guy walks right past the basket or bag or paper, completely oblivious to it, and goes down the stairs empty-handed. I wonder, "How can they not see those things?"

Of course, he didn't get the mental note. Women may want their guys to know what's in their heads without the words having been spoken. Having a conversation about the issues and desired outcomes usually helps—if he's actually listening.

Men have learned to live their entire lives with literal and figurative tunnel vision. They have no trouble simply walking into a room and sitting down— maybe slipping immediately into their "Nothing Box." They may see only the chair, the paper, and an opportunity to take it easy. When and if they want to understand, they can make a conscious effort to "see" the things that need to be done, and take care of them. Motivation is key. Women may need to give them a reason to want to learn to see. Lulabelle's story below provides a good lighthearted example.

Lulabelle—not her real name-- is a mom with a young family who became frustrated when she came home from work very late in the evening to a house full of "assignments." Apparently, she was the only one who knew or cared that they needed to be taken care of before the next day. She was glad to see that her husband had fed the kids, but unhappy that all the evidence was still there to greet her. None of the things that had to be ready for the next day at school were done. The laundry was piled up and "calling" to be washed, dried, and put away.

Frustrated after weeks of the same story, she went on "strike." She stocked corndogs and boxed mac and cheese for the kids' meals, and left her husband to his own creativity for his meals. Only her own laundry and whatever her family had actually placed in the hamper got washed.

It didn't take too many days for her husband to notice that he was running out of clean clothes. She had tried and given up explaining and asking for help, because it wasn't getting results. When he finally asked, she told him the "rules." Clothing in the hamper would be washed, and if he saw them in the washer, he should put them in the dryer, then fold and put them in the bedrooms. Cleaning up the kitchen after meals made her coming home so much more fun.

The next time she worked late, she found a clean kitchen. He was sitting in front of the television with a full laundry basket fresh from the dryer. When she walked into the room, he said, "I'll finish folding these and put them away." She smiled.

Her husband basically said, "Yup! I get it." The strike was over, and things got better for a few months. Every once in a while he gets another reminder, but he notices and responds more quickly. Putting her concerns into words after a "natural consequences" experience led to a win-win solution, and probably some "positive reinforcement" as well.

Practical Tips

It's important to remember that each of us is unique and will respond differently to challenges we face. Generalizing, we know that the male brain responds to movement and prefers systems. They thrive when they have their own space and know they are respected. This means they love to fix things and be on the move, or in their own quiet place where their brains can catch up with their bodies. It's important for women to avoid taking some of men's behavior personally. Their brains may be calling the shots, and it may have nothing to do with the women in their lives.

Put your requests into words, and say it more than once until you know he's heard you. Don't assume he can read your mind. Then, let it go in love rather than resentment and find another way to solve the problem. I know—easier said than done.

Tips for Women in Relationships:

- Cut to the chase. Try to get to the point when communicating with them. Beating around the bush wears them down. Budget your words.
- Appreciation makes them feel loved. "Thank you" goes a long way.
- Give the guys extra time to process emotions.
- Read and respond to his body language. It may give you valuable information.
- Physical affection sometimes communicates better than words.
- Laugh together! It builds connections between your two brains.

The female brain, on the other hand, responds to time spent in relationships, communication, girlfriends, kind words, and compassion. (See chapter 12.)

Tips for Men in Relationships:

- Understand and support their girlfriend relationships. They need each other.
- Loving touch almost always works—hugs, backrubs, foot massages, and wherever it leads.

- Just listen with love and nods when she needs to talk. She isn't looking for a solution. You don't have to "fix" anything here, just let her talk it out for herself.
- Helping in the kitchen and around the house speaks to her heart, as do flowers and "just because" gifts.
- Encourage her creative pursuits without judging the results.
- Appreciate who she is and find ways to let her know.
- Find fun things to enjoy together.

On a personal note, I'm so thankful for my honey of a retired husband who has stepped up to take care of the cooking, gardening, and cleaning that I've not been able to give my usual attention to during this writing process. We each do our own laundry, which works out great. When my friends ask me how that happened, I offer the following explanations. He's an amazing blessing to me, and this book would still be only a dream without his help.

- It was completely his own choice. I had nothing to do with it—well, maybe I did ask for help . . .
- I told him what I needed and didn't assume he could read my mind.
- I let go of the timeline. That part was difficult, but it worked.
- Gratitude helps. Appreciating every helpful gesture brings smiles to both of our faces.
- Complimenting him when we're with friends pays off.

However it happened, we've grown closer, and that feels awesome!

Someone said women marry men hoping they will change, but they don't. And men marry women hoping they won't change, but they do.

As John Gray, author of *Men Are from Mars, Women Are from Venus*, writes, "Men are motivated and empowered when they feel needed . . . . Women are motivated and empowered when they feel cherished."[21]

We've each been given the opportunity to help make someone else's life more pleasant, if we only pay attention. The next two chapters will discuss what that looks like for our fellows, be their friends, family, or someone in need.

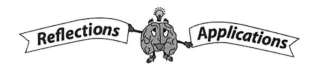

Reflection

Do the differences between your thinking and that of someone of the opposite sex draw you closer or farther apart? Can you change that dynamic?

Application

1. Have a conversation with your partner about things you each appreciate about the other. Notice if that feels comfortable or uncomfortable. Practice makes permanent, not perfect.
2. Can you respect the other person's need to talk or be silent without taking it personally?
3. Are you able to listen without trying to fix the problem?
4. What is most likely to get you laughing together? Try to do more of it!

---

1   Mark Gungor, *"Tale of Two Brains: Unlocking the Secrets to Life, Love, and Marriage ,"* Session I of the DVD series *Laugh Your Way to a Better Marriage,* DVD (Laugh Your Way America, 2005).

2   Jennifer Connellan, Simon Baron-Cohen, Sally Wheelwright, Anna Batki, and Jag Ahluwalia, "Sex Differences in Human Neonatal Social Perception," *Infant Behavior & Development* 23 (January 2000): 113–18, quoted in Leonard Sax, MD, PhD, *Why Gender Matters: What Parents and Teachers Need to Know About the Emerging Science of Sex Differences* (Doubleday, 2005), 19.

3   Leonard Sax, *Why Gender Matters: What Parents and Teachers Need to Know About the Emerging Science of Sex Differences* (Doubleday, 2005), 18–19.

4   Nan Brien, Child Brain Development Consultant to Wisconsin Council on Children and Families, "It Begins In Utero," presentation for the BRAIN Team Gender and Learning conference, Eau Claire, Wisconsin.

5   Sandra Sunquist Stanton, "Gender Friendly Classrooms," presentation for Special Education Council of the Alberta Teachers' Association, Celebrating the Challenges, Kananaskis, Alberta Canada, October 10, 2010.

6   Brien, "It Begins In Utero," presentation.

7   Sax, *Why Gender Matters*, 19–20.

8   Brien, "It Begins In Utero," presentation.

9   Sax, *Why Gender Matters*, 17.

10   Ibid., 15

11 Brien, "It Begins In Utero," presentation.

12 Ibid.

13 Bill and Pam Farrel, *Men Are Like Waffles, Women Are Like Spaghetti: Understanding and Delighting in Your Differences* (Harvest House, 2001), 11.

14 Ibid., 13–14.

15 Ibid., 15.

16 Laugh Your Way to a Better Marriage, http://www.laughyourway.com/about/mark-gungor/.

17 Ibid.

18 Ibid.

19 Ibid.

20 Gary Chapman, *The Five Love Languages: How to Express Heartfelt Commitment to Your Mate* (Northfield Publishing, 1995) 38.

21 John Gray, *Men Are from Mars, Women Are from Venus: A Practical Guide for Improving Communication and Getting What You Want in Your Relationships* (HarperCollins, 1992), 43.

12

FRIENDS, EMPATHY, AND THOSE IN NEED

The meeting of two personalities is like the contact of two chemical substances:
if there is any reaction, both are transformed.
—Carl Gustav Jung

People tend to become more emotionally intelligent as they age and mature.
—Dan Goleman

We've been friends so long—we complete each other's sentences." "How did you know I was about to call you?" Women need each other. It feels so good to be with someone who thinks like you! What happens in the brain to create that connection? What is emotional intelligence and social intelligence? We will explore the answers to these questions, and look closely at empathy and the ways it impacts our relationships with people we know and those who need our help and compassion. First, I'll share a story from my perspective.

When I'm frustrated, relief is at my back door—my neighbor Nancy has the magic touch to help me calm down and deal with any problem. One day I forgot that multitasking seldom ends well. Our dog, Bogey, took off, a container of concentrated juice spilled on the floor, and I couldn't get on the Internet. Uff da!

Then I heard Nancy's voice calling from my backdoor, returning something she had borrowed. Suddenly my major crisis became a minor inconvenience. *I can handle this!*

I remember getting the same boost from our backdoor neighbors when I was growing up. We dropped in on each other with only a knock on the door. Mutual support came along with borrowed sugar, coffee, and sharing big batches of anything we cooked. Friendship makes all the difference, for both mental and physical health.

Nancy and I eventually found Bogey playing with Sage, Nancy's dog and Bogey's best friend. We laughed while cleaning up the sticky mess on my floor. I used her phone to report the network problem. She brightens my day and my life. I'm so grateful, and that's another good thing.[1]

With our busy lives, many of us think we can't make the time for face-to-face contact with close friends. We may connect online, but it's not the same. Texting and e-mails have limited capacity for words, which are only 7 percent of communication. Relying on electronics leaves us missing out on gestures, the emotion that shows in our eyes and expressions, and even the tones and pitch in our voices. Many women feel lonely even in a crowd. Isolation can lead to other problems. Maintaining in-person relationships takes time and effort, but the payback is worth it.

Brain Chemicals and Relationships

Turns out there's an actual physical process at work in our close friendship connections. Did you know being together with longtime close friends sets off changes in our brain and bodies? When you we are present with a dear friend, you might feel a wave of care and appreciation pass through your body. That's the release of a chemical called oxytocin. Friends walking in step, giving hugs, laughing, finishing each other's sentences, and recalling memories they've shared and appreciating each other creates physical changes, which translate into health benefits!

As mentioned earlier, neurotransmitters are the chemicals our brains produce that change the way our brain and body work. Goleman makes several references to the chemical oxytocin in his book *Social Intelligence* when explaining the body and brain's reactions to close personal connections.[2]

So, what actually happens when oxytocin enters our system? "Blood pressure lowers as we slide into the relaxed mode of parasympathetic activity. That shifts metabolism from the ready-to-run large muscle boost of stress arousal to a restorative mode where energy goes into storing nutrients, growth, and healing. Cortisol levels plummet . . . . Our pain threshold rises so that we are less sensitive to discomforts. Even wounds heal faster."[3]

We can give a friend a boost with just a caring touch. Remember that power and use it often. Longfellow's quote says it best, "Ah, how good it feels, the hand of an old friend."

Body/Brain Connections

One of my favorite activities while working in an elementary school was the endless supply of hugs. It's almost impossible to give one without getting one in return. When we are physically close to another person, we each benefit.

Hugs can instantly:

- Boost oxytocin levels, which heals feelings of loneliness, isolation, and anger.
- Lift one's serotonin levels, elevating mood and creating happiness.
- Strengthen the immune system. Gentle pressure on the sternum stimulates the thymus gland, which regulates and balances the body's production of white blood cells, which keep you healthy and disease free.
- Relax muscles. Hugs release tension in the body. Hugs can take away pain; they soothe aches by increasing circulation into the soft tissues.
- Balance the nervous system. The galvanic skin response of someone receiving and giving a hug shows a change in skin conductance. The

effect in moisture and electricity in the skin suggests a more balanced state in the parasympathetic nervous system.

Have you heard that we all need at least four hugs a day? Many people don't get their quota, so ask and offer yours if someone looks like they could use one.

With a Little Help from My Friends

One evening when I was feeling down I made a cup of tea and sat down to read some of my saved greeting cards. One particular handwritten note spoke to me: "We weren't born into this world to see through others, but to see others through." I called my friend Jean, and we met for coffee the next morning and everything looked brighter. Asking for what I needed made more sense than trying to handle it alone. Laughter does heal!

Several years ago, my friend Sharon invited me to join her Tuesday night movie group. We were loosely organized, needing only a phone call to let folks know where we were meeting. When she was diagnosed with a terminal illness, we brought our movie nights to her home with potlucks and videos. She taught us how to live with grace and showed us how to die with love and peace. Our honest and heart wrenching discussions healed all of us in a new way. People moved and the group disbanded after she passed, but we will all remember those times together, laughing, crying, and loving each other.

So go ahead! Enjoy a cup of tea or coffee, a walk along the river, a glass of wine, creative classes, a workout or maybe a road trip with friends. Consider it a prescription for your brain!

A Friendship Comfort Catalogue

During "Supermoms Anonymous," participants generated a "Friendship Comfort Catalogue" of ways they like to connect with their friends.

- Hugs
- Quilting or craft sessions
- Work out together

- A round of golf or tennis game
- A nice, long chatty walk
- "Thrift-saleing" or "Antiquing"
- Movie night
- A freezer meal prep get-together
- There's always shopping . . .
- A bike or horseback ride
- Eating together at home or at another favorite spot
- Enjoying a cup of tea or coffee, or maybe some wine
- Fishing, hunting, the great outdoors
- Mutual back rubs or back scratches
- Give it an extra boost with CHOCOLATE! [4]

Being in the presence of loving friends can help us feel safe and supported, while being alone with our thoughts and our negative self-talk can sometimes tear us apart. Friendship is a gift we give to ourselves and to chosen others in our lives. However, these special connections between people don't always come easily. Each of us has developed our own bundle of filters that can either block or encourage relationships. Our interpretations of social experiences leave us open or closed to others. Successful relationships are the result of skills that social scientists began studying in the 1990s.

The Other Intelligences

Since Alfred Binet first defined and created a way to measure a person's IQ (intelligence quotient), our culture has viewed that as a predictor of success. Dan Goleman was able to shift our focus to other kinds of intelligence through his books *Emotional Intelligence* and *Social Intelligence*. It turns out that self-awareness and an ability to understand and communicate feelings and to draw on them to make sound decisions are equally important. [5] Our learning and accomplishments certainly lead to successful lives, but being able to understand and express our emotions and form meaningful relationships may be much more fulfilling and satisfying.

Emotional Intelligence

Mutually rewarding relationships depend on *emotional intelligence* (EI), a term Dan Goleman coined in his 1995 book by the same name. The brain goes through mental gymnastics to manage the five domains of emotional intelligence:[6]

1. **Knowing one's emotions:** Before we can understand and relate to others, we must first understand our own feelings as they arise or learn in hindsight what was going on for us. We can be blindsided by feelings we don't recognize or understand, leading to bad scenes.

2. **Managing emotions:** When we notice ourselves drifting into anxiety, gloom, worry or irritability, awareness of our feelings can signal us to handle them without making the situation worse. Noting where we hold stress in our bodies can give us a handle to make managing them easier.

3. **Motivating oneself:** When our brains are fully mature—by age thirty or so—we have the capacity to be patient while waiting for something that we would prefer right away. The challenge is choosing to do whatever it takes to get there—eventually. Setting step-by-step goals may not be fun, but the results are often closer to our desired outcomes than impulsive action would be.

4. **Recognizing emotions in others:** Empathy gives us the ability to understand what others are feeling and discern what they might need. Our senses give us a picture of their suffering when we hear their words and pick up on all their nonverbal signs. That triggers similar feelings we've stored as memories.

5. **Handling relationships:** Applying our empathic perception of others' emotions and needs allows us to respond appropriately to them. Over the long term, we can then develop mutually satisfying relationships that grow stronger with time.[7]

Developing our emotional intelligence takes a different sort of learning than most skills. It means paying attention to our own emotions and trying to tune into those of others in our lives. We try to look objectively at our relationships and any patterns we see showing up when we run into problems. Staying open to both positive and negative feedback can help us reach our goals when we are willing to try new ways of connecting with other people.

Social Intelligence

One of my favorite discoveries is that when brain chemicals get into the act, we actually form an interpersonal circuit between our minds! Dan Goleman called this *social intelligence* in his book by the same name.

Goleman presented his perspective on the issues in an interview with *US News and World Report:* "Social intelligence, which is a part of emotional intelligence, refers to our ability to understand and manage relationships. It includes empathy and social skills. Emotional intelligence, in [Goleman's model] . . . includes self-awareness and self-regulation of emotions, and then social intelligence."[8]

Socially successful people instinctively know how to "read" others' emotions through body language, vocal inflection, and other cues.

We constantly broadcast our mental and emotional states, whether we realize it or not. And it works both ways. Has your own mood changed when you're in the presence of someone who is either enthusiastic or morose? Our brains also pick up others' feelings automatically.

Contagious Emotions

Goleman explains, "Moments of contagion represent a remarkable neural event: the formation between two brains of a functional link, a feedback loop that crosses the skin-and-skull barrier between bodies. In systems terms, during this link brains 'couple,' with the output of one becoming input to drive the workings of the other, for the time being forming what amounts to an interbrain circuit. When two entities are connected in a feedback loop as the first changes, so does the second."[9]

So communication with other people goes much deeper than the words we speak or write. Our brains connect directly, but we have to pay attention to our interpretations of those messages. "Social intuition tells us how accurate we are at decoding the stream of nonverbal messages people constantly send, silent modifiers of what they are saying. This steady stream of nonverbal exchanges rushes to and from everyone we interact with, whether in a routine hello or a tense negotiation, transmitting messages received every bit as powerfully as whatever we might be saying. Perhaps *more* powerfully." [10]

So we actually share mutual influence with another person when we're with them. We usually think of empathy as something we share with our close friends, but we also expect professionals we seek help from to have a certain amount of empathy. When we don't feel that connection we might feel disappointed, even though our purpose in seeing them is quite different from the friendship connections.

Empathy and Helping Professions: A Personal Perspective

Growing up, I wanted to help, nurture, and encourage others. My mother often commented to other people that most of my telephone time as a teen was spent listening rather than talking. Our shoe salesman family friend said it was just my big feet. He said they bring me a good understanding. Whatever the source, it felt like a gift that I was called to develop and share. Predictably, that journey led to my counseling career. Listening and caring came easily to me. Students, parents, and staff trusted me with stories of their insurmountable challenges. They needed me to listen and understand, and help them find ways to deal with the things they couldn't change.

Being able to help people started as an answer to prayer. It wasn't long before I found myself going home from school with heavy weights on my shoulders, carrying their stories with me. I had developed "compassion fatigue." Soon, I learned from Fr. John Heagle, our parish priest, the necessity of "learning to care—and not to care." I found that phrase puzzling when he first recommended that I change my approach to counseling for my own mental health. Many in the helping professions need to learn to set emotional boundaries in order to remain helpful to others without sacrificing my own well-being. Fr. Heagle's explanations, examples, and advice got me back on track to be more helpful to others. The degree to which I learned to leave others' issues at school and be present with my family and friends outside school walls determined my own mental health — or burnout.

My experience helped me understand the dilemma others must balance, particularly physicians in medical training. We would like our doctors to provide both technical knowledge and empathy. Let's look at how the brain's normal functioning process makes it an either/or situation.

From the time of our birth, when we see someone in pain, our brain recalls back our own impressions of pain. When that's active, our amygdala (internal homeland security system) sets into motion a chain of signals that disengages our thinking brain, cutting off access to what we've learned.

So we can understand how empathy can interfere with physicians doing their best work for patients. "Bedside manner" sometimes comes up short, because they are remaining focused on providing technical rather than personal support. In a crisis, doctors need to sort through everything they've learned and avoid letting their emotions block access to their thinking brains.

Cool heads are high priority in medical training. Med students are taught to use their thinking brains to put together the best treatment plans for their patients. Unfortunately, that also means sacrificing their natural empathy. Study results show that's exactly what happens. "In one study, about a half of young physicians say their empathy for patients declined over the course of their training (only about a third say it increased)."[11]

Some technical background from Daniel Goleman's book *Focus: The Hidden Driver of Excellence* might help us understand.

Empathy, for most of us, is a positive social skill. When we see someone experiencing a painful or difficult situation, our tendency is to feel it ourselves. Our brains respond as though we ourselves are feeling their pain. For physicians, that would distract them from giving their best care to their patients at a time when they need to focus on the medical procedure instead of the patient's suffering. While most of us want to get away from the painful experience, physicians are trained to block those automatic responses to another person's pain. Jean Decety, professor of psychology and psychiatry at the University of Chicago, did a study that examined physicians' responses, and here's how Goleman explains her findings.

This attentional anesthetic seems to deploy the temporal-parietal junction (or TPJ) and regions of the prefrontal cortex, a circuit that boosts concentration by tuning out emotions. The TPJ protects focus by walling off emotions along with other distractions, and helps keep a distance between oneself and others . . . . The TPJ maneuver insulates the brain from experiencing the wash of emotion—it's the brain basis for the stereotype of someone with cool rationality amid emotional turmoil. A shift into the TPJ mode creates a boundary so you're immune to emotional contagion, freeing your brain from being affected by the other person's emotions while you're focusing.[12]

Recent research shows that empathy helps rather than hurts effectiveness of the doctor/patient relationship. When researchers tried to figure out why patients weren't getting better under the older model, they found that less than half of the patients actually took their meds.[13]

Adding the dimension of empathy made a difference. When the doctor invested the time and attention to make eye contact and listen actively—reflecting what the patient has communicated—patients' motivation increased to follow through with recommendations and take their prescribed medications. Over the course of the treatment relationship, more time was saved than "lost" with empathy.[14]

So, those of us who feel abandoned to technology when our physicians and assistants talk to their computers rather than looking into our eyes will welcome efforts to train doctors in empathy for these important relationships. Wouldn't it be nice if that also improved medical outcomes?

Empathy and Altruism

Everyone has a need to belong, to be seen. We, too, are called to look into another person's eyes. It's easy to be absorbed in our own plans and conversations, ignoring those who are unfamiliar. Eye contact creates a deeper level of communication. When we see others suffering, our memory center brings images of our own suffering. Empathy is activated and spurs us to action. Our world becomes more connected as we respond to others' needs. In our fast-paced world, we can feel invisible. Giving our attention to another person feels good to both of us. As human beings, we're given the "equipment" to relate to other people in ways other creatures can't. Our brains are wired to connect directly with those in our lives.

Dr. Richard Davidson uses a particular test for social sensitivity that shows the level of activity in the fusiform face area when doctors look at a picture of another person's face. Using an fMRI to scan the brain, we can see high levels of activity in that area of the brain in people with high social sensitivity. That brain activity allows them to figure out the feelings of the person in the photo.[15]

Everyone has their own challenges, but if we reach out in love to our companions, we can lighten the load for those who struggle. The people who need us may be closer than we think. Altruism is good for the soul. We can certainly share what we have and the personal gifts we've been given.

Elizabeth Ann Seton said, "Choose to live simply, in order that others may simply live." [16] Listening and seeing God in the face of those we meet every day brings us closer to him and each other.

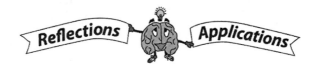

Reflection
Think of a time when you and a good friend said volumes to each other with only a look shared between you.

Application
1. If you were able to give your younger self some friendship advice, what would you say?
2. Let a friend who's able to know what you're thinking, or finish your sentences, know how much you appreciate that connection.
3. Expand your horizons. Try to learn something new from someone outside your usual circle of friends.

1   Sandra Sunquist Stanton, "Sisterhood Is Powerful: Brain Boost from Friendship," *Queen of the Castle Magazine*, July 2014, 29.

2   Goleman, *Social Intelligence: The Revolutionary New Science of Human Relationships* (Bantam, 2006), 164, 202–3, 216.

3   Ibid., 243.

4   Supermoms Anonymous Group, "Sisterhood Is Powerful," *Queen of the Castle Magazine*, July 2014, 29.

5   Goleman, *Social Intelligence*, 243.

6   Daniel Goleman, *Emotional Intelligence: Why It Can Matter More than IQ* (Bantam Books, 1995), 43.

7   Ibid.

8   Daniel Goleman as quoted by Deborah Kotz, "Straight-A Students, Take Note: Your Emotional Intelligence May Mean More to Your Success Than Book Smarts," *Secrets of Your Brain* (US News & World Report, 2011), 33.

9   Goleman, *Social Intelligence*, 39-40.

10   Goleman, *Focus: The Hidden Driver of Excellence* (HarperCollins, 2013), 116.

11   Tim Ryan, *A Mindful Nation* (Hay House, 2012) and Jeffrey Sachs, *The Price of Civilization* (Random House, 2013) as quoted in Dan Goleman, *Focus: The Hidden Driver of Excellence* (HarperCollins, 2013), 113.

12   Goleman, *Focus*, 110–11.

13   Adapted, Goleman, *Focus*, 112.

14   Goleman, *Focus*, 115.

15   Ibid., 117.

16   Elizabeth Ann Seton quoted in John Heagle, *Justice Rising: The Emerging Biblical Vision* (Orbis Books, 2010), 160.

13 THE GIFT OF FAMILY

Other things may change us, but we start and end with the family.
—Anthony Brandt

So far, we've talked about taking care of ourselves and our friendships. God has also called us to be his hands and feet for those he has given to us to love. Families are a long-term gift from God through which the youngest to the oldest receive the nurturing they need. This is the place where our hearts and hopes live and grow. Here we find the best and the worst of ourselves and our family members, and learn to love them even when we sometimes may not like them very much.

Families provide history, memories, and challenges for our brains. In this chapter, we will look at roles families play in developing the mind and caring for our children and disabled family members, young and old, when they need us most.

You've probably heard the "nature versus nurture" brain development debate. Both nature and nurture are very important throughout our lives. We know that *nature* comes first, in the form of our 100 billion brain cells. Human babies' brains are not fully developed at birth. That's why we need our families to *nurture* our bundle of neurons, creating experiences making it possible for them to work together. Growing minds grow best within the safety and care of loving families. At this stage of our lives, our children may have given us wonderful opportunities to watch children's miraculous brains grow at astonishing rates.

Grandchildren—Pure Joy!

If I had known grandchildren would be this much fun, I would have had them first! They tug at our hearts and leave us laughing uncontrollably as we watch and listen to them making sense of their world. We often wish we would have written down all their comments and the spontaneous things they do, surprising us into joy. Here are a few stories to illustrate:

Grandpa Mike has a favorite tradition with his six-year-old grandson, Jameson. They've gone out for breakfast almost every Friday morning since the little guy could walk, so they've gotten to know the staff well. The pair likes to race each other to the restaurant door. Two weeks ago, Jameson won. He burst through the doors, threw his arms into the air, and announced, "She's here! She's here!"

"Who's here?" the hostess asked. Big smiles and laughs.

"My sister's here! She's born!" Jameson trumpeted.

At their table, he couldn't wait until their regular waitress arrived. The moment he spotted her, he stood on the seat and shouted, "My sister's here! My sister's born! And she's even cuter than me!"

The other diners couldn't help but hear him. Mike noticed many smiles and appreciative laughter.

Children's impressions of their world are a constant source for surprise and humor. Their literal interpretations give us a fresh look at our own world. Here's another story to illustrate:

Grandma Diane thought it might be fun to get some cute dinosaur-shaped snacks for her grandkids. Sitting down with them for a snack, she tasted one herself, and made an awful face! "These are awful! They taste like cardboard!" Four-year-old grandson Arthur looked quizzically at her, then at the snack in his hand and thought for a few seconds. Then he asked, "Grandma, when did you eat cardboard?"

A third story illustrates another point. Sometimes our reactions can compromise our important relationship with our grandchildren's parents—our children. Lorena announced the birth of her first granddaughter and shared photos. She told us about the first time she held the precious baby. She told her son, "This is my little girl!" He reminded her, "She's my little girl. She's your granddaughter." That can be a tough boundary for grandparents, but it's worth mentioning so that all three generations can enjoy each other.

As first-time grandparents, we have to learn how different that role is from our earlier parenting. Keeping up with the little ones wears out our bodies, but fills our hearts with joy. Listening and loving are more important now than directing and offering unsolicited advice. We know they could benefit from our experience and the mistakes that we now recognize, but that learning must go through their own brains. If they ask, we can go ahead and share our experience. If not, our job is simply to love, appreciate, and encourage them.

Nurturing Grandchildren's Brains and Relationships

So when we're able to spend time with those little bundles of energy, where do we start? Lucky grandparents may be able to play with them weekly. Others may have to rely on electronic communication—FaceTime or Skype for a visual connection. Maybe we have only the postal service. In any case, *Grandloving: Making Memories with Your Grandchildren* offers more than two hundred activities to add to our already deep well of activity experience. A comment from the introduction makes a valuable point:

"Praise is like a puppy's kisses—a few licks on the cheek are the best thing ever, but more is soon overwhelming."[1] Grandchildren benefit most from specific and limited praise. "Please tell me about your picture." "I like the way your blue and red come together to make purple." "Does the picture have a story? What happened before and after this picture?" These comments require our full attention and create connections between us, as opposed to the much easier and overused, "That's great, honey!"[2] I had to bite my tongue when that one came out of my mouth. Habits are hard to break, even when we know a better way. Good thing we can keep learning!

Grandparents as Parents

Increasingly, and for a variety of reasons, grandparents find themselves back in their parenting role, responsible for the primary care of their grandchildren. Fortunately, resources on child development have improved since we raised our own family. Grandparents are frequent participants in our Building Baby's Brain classes, and Eau Claire's Grandparents as Parents group also meets regularly to support them. We'd like to make the most of those crucial early years, so here's a brief summary of what their rapidly developing brains need.

Babies' experiences during their first years set the foundation for the rest of their lives. The brain connections formed during their first years really do last forever. They need to feel safe and able to impact their world. These brain basics can be helpful for anyone who cares for infants:

- Babies depend on their parents and caregivers to give them the experiences that will connect their 100 billion brain cells. They are only 25 percent wired together at birth. Until they are connected to each other, these cells can't accomplish anything.
- To help us understand developing brain connections, we can compare the brain's wiring to a telephone connection from Chicago to Minneapolis. Placing the call with a wiring system like a baby's immature set of brain connections would make the target phone ring—along with most of the rest of them in the city. When we call the same "phone number" again and again, that path becomes stronger and more refined. In the brain, experience and repetition strengthens the specific series of connections allowing the "call" to reach the intended "receiver" without any other numbers responding. Think about babies' fascination discovering their fingers and toes. They are just learning that they can control their "brand new toys." What fun to have them attached to their bodies!

- Face-to-face time together with adult caregivers gives each child an opportunity to study facial expressions, learn about emotions and the basics of forming relationships. Attachment is essential for the child's mental health. And it's so much fun!
- Tummy time is also crucial to develop their core, neck, and shoulder muscles, and their vestibular systems. It builds foundation for balance with strong muscles.
- Children need to view the world as a safe place. If exposed to toxic situations, their mental energy is consumed trying to avoid pain. When they feel safe, they are free to develop brain foundations for language, emotional development, or relationship skills.

The following eight easy-reference tips created by the Brain Research Awareness Information Network (BRAIN Team) are included in the Baby Brain Bags provided for parents and grandparents at the Building Baby's Brain classes.

Eight Gifts Every Child's Brain Needs:

1. **Security:** You create his world. If he feels safe, he will be willing to try new things. If he is fearful, he may withdraw, refuse contact, and choose to protect himself.
2. **Touch:** Loving touch soothes the central nervous system for both you and your child. It communicates safety and love. Enjoy snuggles, massage, and rocking while reading to her. These times are short.
3. **Healthy food:** His brain doesn't store the fuel it needs to operate. An infant's brain uses 70 percent of his body's energy. Every day it needs water, fresh fruit, and omega-3 healthy fats. These building blocks create and strengthen connections between his 100 billion brain cells.
4. **Music:** Both sides of her brain are active when she enjoys music. It's a workout for her brain. She forms stronger memories when many parts of the brain are involved.
5. **Movement:** Every time your child moves, his brain and body work together, getting stronger. Play together! Dance, skip, clap, and let him help you in the kitchen and garden. His learning becomes

multidimensional, richer, and easier for him to remember and build on as he grows.

6. **Reading and language:** For many children, sitting quietly and reading together is their favorite activity—especially before bed. Time with you helps them learn language patterns and how to form relationships. Does reading the same book over and over again get old? Remember repetition is exactly what their brains need to learn.

7. **Rest and sleep:** During quiet times her brain gets a chance to process her mountain of recent experiences. When she's busy, her neurons are taking in sensory information. Her brain's original cells still need to be connected to one another. That happens during these breaks.

8. **You!**

Enjoy time together often and as long as your child shows an interest. Let her teach you what works best for her. Electronic media may be convenient, but it cannot substitute for person-to-person interaction with you. She learns that she matters when you respond to her. Enjoy this together time and make some memories.[3]

Brain and relationship building activities don't need to cost a bundle to be effective. School-age children may stretch our creativity and energy, but they also need an adult who offers them unconditional love and acceptance.

Connecting with Older Grandkids

Whenever we spend time with the children in our lives, we are helping them understand and manage their feelings and relationships. Knowing they have our undivided attention also helps build their ability to trust. The children's relationship skills may be compromised by extensive reliance on electronics for communication. Grandparents may have golden opportunities to counteract that in our grandkids. Here are some ways to make that happen:

- Let them teach you one of their favorite hands-on activities.
- Walking, working, or playing side by side generates good conversation.
- Car time with just the two of you makes for easy conversation.

- Doing something together side by side often works great.
- Try cooking or a board game.
- Ask questions that can't be answered with yes or no. Try "Tell me about`. . .`"
- Some kids might like to choose and tell you about the best and worst parts of the day/week. We call this "High-Low."[4]

We never know what our grandchildren's brains will choose to hold on to, but making memories is so much fun! Giving them and all family members our full attention when they feel like talking can take relationships to a higher level. Give mindful listening a try.

Mindful Listening

Fully focused listening has been called the greatest gift one person can give another. Mindfulness is the opposite of multitasking. When listening mindfully, we give our full attention to the speaker, their body language, the tone of their voice, and any changes in their movement or skin tone. Our brains are completely tuned in to both their words and the unspoken content that is often even more "true." On the other hand, dividing our attention between the person we're listening to and another task gives us an incomplete picture. We've all experienced a conversation with someone whose mind is somewhere else. We've probably caught ourselves doing the same thing. It's all too common to use our mental energy planning what we will say when they take a breath, rather than actually processing what they are saying. The person we're listening to gets the unspoken message that neither they nor their thoughts matter. Truly listening is hard work! Attending with our ears, eyes, and possibly caring touch takes significant effort, but the speaker feels heard, encouraged, and validated.

Communication experts suggest that we listen carefully without interrupting, then check to see if we understood correctly the feelings they've expressed: "It sounds like you felt sad, angry, excited . . ." In case we missed the mark interpreting their complete message, this gives them a chance to clarify what they've said. Genuine interest as they restate their experience usually leads to growing trust, more sharing, and a deepening relationship. Both friends and family deserve this special attention and our care and respect. Listening is only one part of the role of caregiver for family members with a disability.

Caring for Young Disabled Family Members

Family members of all ages need to be heard and valued. This is especially true of those who are dealing with a disability.

Helping parents understand and accept their children's disabilities was one of the most difficult parts of my school counseling. Each parent had dreams for their child, and usually feared hearing the assessment results. "Welcome to Holland" is an analogy parents use to illustrate their own reactions. They had been looking forward to all the markers of successful development much like planning a trip. Let's say they thought they were headed for Italy for a wonderful vacation. Then the plane began its descent to the airport, and the pilot announced, "Welcome to Holland, everyone. Enjoy your stay!" Then protests were heard. They began painfully grieving their rerouted dreams. "I didn't sign up for this! I thought we were going to Italy! I don't know anything about this country!" They needed support and time to grieve, much the same as anyone experiencing the loss of a loved one. Each person gathered up their life experience, which determined how they dealt with their news. Acceptance or denial. Sometimes, difficult choices created enormous challenges for relationships among family members and collaboration with the school.

Managing the situation became somewhat easier when they were able to find joy in their "Holland" experience, learn and apply appropriate expectations for their child's development, and communicate openly with educators. Many found support in talking with other parents who truly understood. They learned from each other's successes. Some added music to their lives in new ways and found that it healed both the child's and parents' spirits.

Caring for an Aging Disabled Adult

We seldom feel adequately prepared to become the caregiver for a spouse or aging parent. When we find ourselves in a role reversal—parenting our parents — it's important to seek information and support from reliable sources when making a plan both for their care and for our own mental health. The American Association of Retired Persons website offers suggestions for the planning that will be necessary in the following areas:

- Ask for what you need. Planning and Resources
- Benefits and Insurance
- Legal and Money Matters
- Providing Care
- Senior Housing
- End of Life Care
- Grief and Loss[5]

Check online and with local agencies for information and actual physical support for your family member. They seldom have a substantial marketing budget, so other people in your same situation may be able to help you find services that fit your unique situation. Kindred spirits will also be better able to understand and help you feel supported. In the meantime, your own creativity might lead you to some tools you have right at home—like music! Switch to senses.

Senses Are Keys to Support Memory for Ailing Elderly

When our elderly family members are unable to care for themselves, we do whatever we can to make their lives easier and more pleasant. We know what to do to help them physically, even if they can't understand why they must make a move to another home.

Accessing the brain at any age involves the senses, through which every bit of information enters the organ. Looking back at when we formed our lifelong memories, music was often a defining element of the years when we established social connections and made important life decisions. Our memories are linked to the popular music of that time. Those memories, having earned a place in our elderly relatives' brains for their lifetime, can make retrieving them easier for caregivers.

When memory issues complicate the problem, more complicated interventions may be necessary. Lee Anna Rasar's presentation "Cracking the Dementia Code—Music and Memories" suggests ways that music and our senses can help access their memories across six dimensions: Motor, Cognitive, Language, Social, Emotional, and Spiritual.

- Motor: Pairing dance and movement with musical activities can improve their range of motion, decrease tremors, and help them keep a steady beat to rhythm patterns, helping them access part of their motor memory.

- Cognitive: When they originally formed memories with music, many parts of the brain were involved. Matching imagery to music with motion provides a context for retrieving memories. For example, a song about wringing out a dishrag reminds them of a familiar activity. Recalling that encourages them to rotate their wrists and exercise those muscles.

- Language: Putting language to music often makes it easier to remember. The two together can help draw their attention to an object or spot in the room, or move in a certain way or do something else they've been asked to do. Singing games engage their attention and enthusiasm when straight language might not.

- Social: Music can be used to redirect their negative responses to situations, using tempo, dynamics, and musical form. Life review activities go smoothly when we sing or play familiar songs from their youth.

- Emotional: Music can help manage their moods. Choose calming—possibly baroque—music to encourage relaxation or energizing music to boost activity levels. Remembering each person's memories are paired with unique emotions, it's important to be flexible in case their memories of that particular song are uncomfortable ones.

- Spiritual: Many elderly have strong emotional ties to religious music. Encouraging them to sing or listen to them will probably evoke memories of situations they like to recall and talk about.[6]

Music supports memory retrieval, but other sensory experiences are also helpful. A warm footbath and massage helps circulation and is soothing for most people. Hugs, when welcome, bring people a sense of closeness.

Many sensory activities are pictured and described on Pinterest to give you some ideas. Hanging old CDs in a sunny window creates wonderful rainbows around the room. Kinetic sand available at craft stores feels great in the hands when carefully introduced. Exploring fruit visually, identifying it by scent or only through touch can be fun. Watching birds or spending time in nature often helps body and spirit. Sharing photos in whatever form may bring pleasant memories to their attention. Videotape the stories so you don't lose them. Our elderly relatives have a treasure trove to share. Unlimited possibilities are out there, but the best ones involve family members of all ages showing love to one another.

We want to take the best care possible of our family members, but it's an intense and demanding commitment. One of the best things you can do for them is to take care of yourself.

Caring for the Caregiver

According to a pamphlet from the Eau Claire County Aging and Disability Center, about one-fourth of adults are caregivers. They do not have to live with the person to be a caregiver; many fill the role while living at a distance.[7] Paying attention to the signs of stress and taking steps to relieve it can offset both physical and psychological problems. They creep up on us gradually, so it helps to have someone help you monitor your own possibly compromised immune function, blood pressure, gastrointestinal problems, and other body issues. Depression, anxiety, anger, sadness, changes in eating and sleeping habits, difficulty concentrating, social withdrawal, and other psychological signs point to a need for support and relief.[8]

Many people feel more able to manage the challenges when they find someone in a similar situation to trust, talking and listening to each other. Rest for your own body and brain is very important in keeping yourself strong. Aging and Disability offices may be able to provide information to help you give respite care for your family member so you can take a break and restore your energy.

Think about the activities that build you up, the things that light up your life, and try to find a way to include them in your routine.

Caregiving is so *daily*! As a caregiver, your days can be a series of consuming urgencies as your family member makes demands that you are unable to meet. You might try making a list of activities that restore your spirit—a Comfort Catalogue—and keep it handy for unexpected opportunities when someone asks if they can help. To get you started, here's a list of ideas:

- Time with friends
- A solitary walk
- A cuddly blanket or jacket
- Some fresh flowers
- A cup of coffee, tea, or hot chocolate
- Fresh fruit
- A massage—foot, chair, or body
- Favorite music—relaxing or energizing
- Connecting with a special friend on the phone
- Reviewing a collection of favorite greeting cards
- Scripture
- A hot bath
- Exercise
- A favorite magazine
- Old movies
- Watching favorite old comedy shows
- Sleeping in
- Gardening
- Sitting in a sunny window[9]

You get the idea. Sometimes when we most need comfort, our brains may be least likely to be able to access our internal list. It's easier to just pick it up and read what you've written.

Be sure to ask for what you need. It's not selfish. It will make both your life and that of your family member more pleasant and satisfying. Please trust someone else with your feelings. Prayer gives many a sense of peace. Keeping a gratitude list might help you focus on and increase the positive moments in your days.

Our families are indeed where we start and finish. Our experiences with them probably hold both the peaks and valleys of our lives. They bring us a special brand of love, joy, and pain that God can use to make us more like him. Gratitude transforms our memories of the journey and relationships. Thank God for giving us families to nurture us and develop our strong brains.

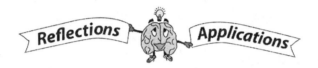

Reflection

Who became "God with skin on" for you? Did you have someone who brought safety and unconditional love to your spirit? Can you recognize God's provision and how he has loved you through them?

Application

1. Journal about your journey, those who love you, and those who accept your love. Maybe have a "heart-to-heart" to let them know you've seen God work through them. Putting it into words somehow makes it more real for both of you.

2. God carries us in our toughest times. Recall what God taught you through a major struggle. Can you be thankful for anything that came out of that time in your life?

3. Mine your collection of old and more recent photographs for memories. Share those stories with family members and invite them to share their own. Try videotaping the sessions to create still another treasure.

---

1 Sue Johnson and Julie Carlson, *Grandloving: Making Memories with Your Grandchildren* (Heartstrings Press, 2000), 1.

2 Ibid., 1.

3   "Brain Research Awareness Information Network, *Dr. Brain's Basic 8*, series of pamphlets (BRAIN Team, Eau Claire, Wisconsin, 2006).

4   Sandra Sunquist Stanton, "Back to School Brain Tips," *Queen of the Castle Magazine*, September 2014, 34.

5   AARP, Caregiving Resource Center website, http://www.aarp.org/home-family/caregiving/providing-care/.

6   Lee Anna Rasar, "Cracking the Dementia Code: Music and Memories," presentation, May 5, 2014.

7   Mardi Richmond (writer), Eva Bernstein (designer), Meg Biddle (illustrator), "50 Things Every Caregiver Should Know," pamphlet, (Journeyworks Publishing, 2003).

8   Massachusetts General Hospital, "Identifying Caregiver Stress," *Mind, Mood & Memory*, April 2011, 3.

9   Supermoms Anonymous Group, "Personal Comfort Catalogue," collected from group, Putnam Heights Elementary School, May, 2000.

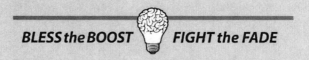

BLESS the BOOST   *FIGHT the FADE*

Bless the Boost and Fight the Fade: Your Relationships

Bless the Boost
- Wisdom: Our ability to gather information and offer insights based on experience stays with us and may even improve with time.[1] With maturity, many of us are better able to direct our attention and energy toward the issues that we can change and let go of the others.
- Acceptance: Many long-term friendships have shown us strengths and weaknesses are a complete package. Appearances may be less important than helping others. We might find it easier to appreciate ourselves and others, quirks included.

Fight the Fade
- Source memory: Where did I park my car? Which restaurant was that? When did we eat there? Can you help me find my keys? Retrieving information from source memory gets more difficult as we get older.[2] Triggering as many senses as possible can make that easier. Visualize, write it down, say it out loud, or take a photo, whatever works. If none of those help, relax your brain and give yourself some time. It'll come to you.
- Multitasking: Shifting our attention quickly between two or more activities means less brainpower devoted to each of them—at any age. That gets even harder as we get older.[3] Consciously sticking with only one thing at a time will result in better outcomes.

---

1   Nelson with Gilbert, Achieving Optimal Memory, 52.

2   Ibid., 51.

3   Ibid.

Part V
WHAT'S NEXT?

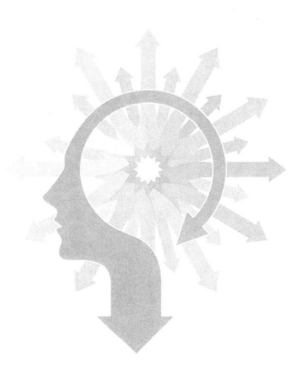

Max Your Mind

REFLECTIONS AND APPLICATIONS

When a book comes to an end, it feels sad sometimes, like a relationship is over. Thank you, reader, for joining this journey to understand and make the most of our incredible God-created brains. Knowing that they continue to grow and change might convince us to make those changes positive rather than negative. Appreciating the "Boost" and dealing with the "Fade" that comes with passing years are keys to a full and satisfying life.

If I had to choose one word for the purpose of *Max Your Mind*, it would probably be *hope*. Our friend Mary is an inspiration in this regard. She is making a miraculous recovery from a life-threatening vehicle accident just over two years ago. She and her husband are living testaments to hope and the benefits of prayer and hard work in the face of impossible odds after her serious brain injury. My husband and I are in awe of their strength and courage as they trust us with their stories of struggles and successes. Their hope inspires positive action for me and for each of us as we face daily choices to support our own brain health with exercise, nutrition, love, laughter, time with caring family, friends, and activities that light up our brains. Now, I plan to follow Bob Goff's challenge to "Go do

189

stuff!" I invite you to do the same, create your own brain boost stories and share them with me.

I've gathered the Reflections and Applications from each of the previous thirteen chapters into this section to make it easier for you to pull together your thoughts now that you've read *Max Your Mind*. It might be a helpful guide for review whether or not you chose to take personal notes while you read. Thanks for sharing this journey with me!

Part I: The Brain

Chapter 1: What Lights up Your Brain?
Reflection
Do you believe God created you with special gifts? They are blessings from God to bring satisfaction and joy to your life and the lives of others.
Application
1. List three things you were "made" to do.
2. As a neurobics exercise, share a meal with family or friends with the radio, TV, cell phones, and all other electronic devices turned off. Focus your attention on your conversation and the taste and texture of the food.
3. Discuss any differences between the electronic-free meal and your usual dining experience.

Chapter 2: Brain Basics
Reflection
Our God-created human brain is the most complex organism in the world. What part or brain function would you like to learn more about?
Application
1. How do you prefer to receive information? Is it easiest for you to read, listen, talk with others about it, write about it, or learn hands-on (kinesthetically)?

2. How are you most comfortable passing that information on to other people? Our favorite paths are often our most effective ones.

3. Teaching someone else what you've learned is a great way to lock the learning in your memory. Explain parts of brain function to someone else.

Chapter 3: Memories under Construction
Reflection
Have you ever forgotten why you came into a room? Are you able to laugh about it without judging yourself or panicking about losing your mind?
Application

1. How do you deal with Event Boundary? What helps you keep your intention in mind when moving from one room to another?

2. Recall an event that seems different to you now than when it first happened. Discuss the changes in this memory package with another person who shared the original experience with you.

3. Can you recall your brain going blank when you were fearful or upset? Think about your amygdala—internal security system—and the "protection" it provides. Sometimes we might want to let our executive function—the prefrontal cortex—calm it down so we will be able to function.

Part II: The Body

Chapter 4: Your Body as Stress Buster
Reflection
Pause to consider and be thankful for each part of your body that is working properly. What an amazing creation!
Application

1. How do your mind, body, and spirit respond to focused breathing? Are the centering exercises helpful for your mental and emotional well-being?

2. Choose a person, place, or experience that you can focus on in order to bring your mind into peace and serenity. Take three deep belly breaths with this loving image in your mind. Practice this daily, and notice if it helps you with stress.

3. Try journaling to clarify your own thoughts and feelings, then revisit what you've written a month later to notice if the insights you wrote are helpful over time.

Chapter 5: Input for Output

Reflection

Our bodies always try to communicate what they need. Have you ever gotten a headache when you forgot to drink enough water? Have you noticed any other warning signs?

Application

1. How does your mind and body let you know what they need? How do you respond?

2. What would you like to add to or drop from your nutritional habits? What is your plan for making that happen?

3. Try reducing the amount of added sugar you consume. Note how your body responds after a week or so.

Chapter 6: Move It!

Reflection

What type of exercise works best for you? What obstacles threaten to keep you from being active? Can you deal with obstacles that get in the way?

Application

1. Choose a workout that you and a friend can enjoy together, encouraging each other to follow through on that important goal.

2. List ways to overcome each obstacle that you listed in the reflections.

3. Some people notice that working out affects mind, body, or spirit. Do you see any changes in your memory, your ability to think clearly, or your ability to relax?

Part III: The Spirit

Chapter 7: Connecting with God through Prayer
Reflection

Recall a situation during which you felt particularly close to God. What was going on in your life? Was it an easy or challenging time for you? How would you describe your feelings about this special connection with him? What was the outcome for you and for your faith?

Application

1. Each of us has a unique style for connecting with God. Which type of prayer "feeds" your soul?
2. Has God ever let you know that he wanted you to take some action? How did he get your attention? How did you respond?
3. How did you feel about the situation after following or not following his guidance?

Chapter 8: Gratitude and Trust
Reflection

1. Reflect on the influence of gratitude, trust, and love or fear on your well-being.
2. Recall a circumstance when you were unable to think clearly or remember what actually happened while you were fearful.
3. How does your body feel when you appreciate someone else or they express appreciation for something you've done for them?

Application

Create your own Blessings Basket or Gratitude List:

1. Find a decorative box or basket.
2. Get colored index cards, with at least enough of each color for the days of the week for an entire month.
3. Scope out your blessings during the day. Your plan to write them down will help you keep your focus, and you'll notice more every day.

4. Record as many blessings as you can on the card. The trick is to notice new ones, trying to avoid repeating them. You might begin with three to five and increase from there.
5. During bleak days, reread some of the cards to re-experience your positive memory.
6. www.aHolyExperience.com has endless suggestions for you to choose from to creatively tailor your own Gratitude List.

Chapter 9: Humor Does a Body Good
Reflection
Recall events when belly laughs made you breathless. How did you feel afterwards?
Application
1. Try Laughter Yoga!
2. Think of an incident when you felt better after a good laugh.
3. Come up with things to help you laugh as much as a child. How many laughs can you pack into one day? Can you make it to 400?
4. Thank someone who makes you laugh. Find a creative way to let them know they are supporting your health.

Chapter 10: Music Makes Your Spirit Sing!
Reflection
How does music affect your mood, learning, and activity level?
Application
1. List your go-to recording artists for "oldies," workout, worship, and relaxation music.
2. What recording artists bring back favorite memories for you?
3. Remember learning the alphabet song? Are you able to recall anything else that you learned in a musical format?

Part IV: Relationships

Chapter 11: Gender Matters

Reflection

Do the differences between your thinking and that of someone of the opposite sex draw you closer or farther apart? Can you change that dynamic?

Application

1. Have a conversation with your partner about things you each appreciate about the other. Notice if that feels comfortable or uncomfortable. Practice makes permanent, not perfect.
2. Can you respect the other person's need to talk or be silent without taking it personally?
3. Are you able to listen without trying to fix the problem?
4. What is most likely to get you laughing together? Try to do more of it!

Chapter 12: Friends, Empathy, and Those in Need

Reflection

Think of a time when you and a good friend said volumes to each other with only a look shared between you.

Application

1. If you were able to give your younger self some friendship advice, what would you say?
2. Let a friend who's able to know what you're thinking, or finish your sentences, know how much you appreciate that connection.
3. Expand your horizons. Try to learn something new from someone outside your usual circle of friends.

Chapter 13: The Gift of Family

Reflection

Who became "God with skin on" for you? Did you have someone who brought safety and unconditional love to your spirit? Can you recognize God's provision and how he has loved you through them?

Application

1. Journal about your journey, those who love you, and those who accept your love. Maybe have a "heart-to-heart" to let them know you've seen God work through them. Putting it into words somehow makes it more real for both of you.

2. God carries us in our toughest times. Recall what God taught you through a major struggle. Can you be thankful for anything that came out of that time in your life?

3. Mine your collection of old and more recent photographs for memories. Share those stories with family members and invite them to share their own. Try videotaping the sessions to create still another treasure.

RESOURCES FOR MEMORY LOSS AND ALZHEIMER'S DISEASE

This book presents only general information about brain health. If you are looking for more detailed diagnostics to help your family member, please consult your physician or the many reliable resources available online, including the Alzheimer's Association (http://www.alz.org/national/documents/checklist_10signs.pdf).

Special thanks to the Alzheimer's Association for their permission to include the following checklist and typical behaviors to help readers find their best ways to help family members:

Have you noticed any of these warning signs?

Please list any concerns you have and take this sheet with you to the doctor.

Note: This list is for information only and not a substitute for a consultation with a qualified professional.

1. **Memory loss that disrupts daily life.** One of the most common signs of Alzheimer's, especially in the early stages, is forgetting recently learned information. Others include forgetting important dates or events, asking

for the same information over and over, and relying on memory aides (e.g., reminder notes or electronic devices) or family members for things they used to handle on their own.

What's typical? Sometimes forgetting names or appointments, but remembering them later.

2. **Challenges in planning or solving problems.** Some people may experience changes in their ability to develop and follow a plan or work with numbers. They may have trouble following a familiar recipe or keeping track of monthly bills. They may have difficulty concentrating and take much longer to do things than they did before.

What's typical? Making occasional errors when balancing a checkbook.

3. **Difficulty completing familiar tasks at home, at work, or at leisure.** People with Alzheimer's often find it hard to complete daily tasks. Sometimes, people may have trouble driving to a familiar location, managing a budget at work, or remembering the rules of a favorite game.

What's typical? Occasionally needing help to use the settings on a microwave or to record a television show.

4. **Confusion with time or place.** People with Alzheimer's can lose track of dates, seasons, and the passage of time. They may have trouble understanding something if it is not happening immediately. Sometimes they may forget where they are or how they got there.

What's typical? Getting confused about the day of the week but figuring it out later.

5. **Trouble understanding visual images and spatial relationships.** For some people, having vision problems is a sign of Alzheimer's. They may have difficulty reading, judging distance, and determining color or contrast. In terms of perception, they may pass a mirror and think someone else is in the room. They may not recognize their own reflection.

What's typical? Vision changes related to cataracts.

6. **New problems with words in speaking or writing.** People with Alzheimer's may have trouble following or joining a conversation.

They may stop in the middle of a conversation and have no idea how to continue or they may repeat themselves. They may struggle with vocabulary, have problems finding the right word or call things by the wrong name (e.g., calling a watch a "hand clock").

What's typical? Sometimes having trouble finding the right word.

7. **Misplacing things and losing the ability to retrace steps.** A person with Alzheimer's disease may put things in unusual places. They may lose things and be unable to go back over their steps to find them again. Sometimes, they may accuse others of stealing. This may occur more frequently over time.

What's typical? Misplacing things from time to time, such as a pair of glasses or the remote control.

8. **Decreased or poor judgment.** People with Alzheimer's may experience changes in judgment or decision-making. For example, they may use poor judgment when dealing with money, giving large amounts to telemarketers. They may pay less attention to grooming or keeping themselves clean.

What's typical? Making a bad decision once in a while.

9. **Withdrawal from work or social activities.** A person with Alzheimer's may start to remove themselves from hobbies, social activities, work projects, or sports. They may have trouble keeping up with a favorite sports team or remembering how to complete a favorite hobby. They may also avoid being social because of the changes they have experienced.

What's typical? Sometimes feeling weary of work, family, and social obligations.

10. **Changes in mood and personality.** The mood and personalities of people with Alzheimer's can change. They can become confused, suspicious, depressed, fearful, or anxious. They may be easily upset at home, at work, with friends, or in places where they are out of their comfort zone.

What's typical? Developing very specific ways of doing things and becoming irritable when a routine is disrupted.

If you have questions about any of these warning signs, the Alzheimer's Association recommends consulting a physician. Early diagnosis provides the best opportunities for treatment, support, and future planning.

For more information, go to alz.org/10signs or call 800.272.3900.

LOOKING FOR MORE?

Amen, Daniel G. *Use Your Brain to Change Your Age: Secrets to Look, Feel, and Think Younger Every Day.* Crown, 2012.

Andreasen, Nancy C. *The Creating Brain: The Neuroscience of Genius.* Dana Press, 2005.

Arden, John B. *Rewire Your Brain: Think Your Way to a Better Life.* Wiley, 2010.

Baron-Cohen, Simon. *The Essential Difference: The Truth about the Male & Female Brain.* Basic Books, 2003.

Beauregard, Mario, and Denyse O'Leary. *The Spiritual Brain: A Neuroscientist's Case for the Existence of the Soul.* Harper One, 2007.

Bombeck, Erma. *Forever, Erma: Best-Loved Writing from America's Favorite Humorist.* Andrews and McMeel, 1996.

Brien, Nan. "Great Beginnings: The First Years Last Forever." Presentation and pamphlet series. Wisconsin Council on Children and Families, 2000.

Cameron, Julia. *The Artist's Way: A Spiritual Path to Higher Creativity.* Tarcher/Perigree, 1992.

Childre, Doc. *Freeze Frame: One Minute Stress Management, A Scientifically Proven Technique for Clear Decision Making and Improved Health.* Planetary Publications, 1998.

Davidson, Richard, and Sharon Begley. *The Emotional Life of Your Brain: How Its Unique Patterns Affect the Way You Think, Feel, and Live—and How You Can Change Them.* Hudson Street, 2012.

Dennison, Paul and Gail. *Brain Gym.* Edu-Kinesthetics, 1986.
    Brain Gym: Teacher's Edition. Edu-Kinesthetics, 1989.

Doidge, Norman. *The Brain That Changes Itself: Stories of Personal Triumph from the Frontiers of Brain Science.* Penguin Books, 2007.

Farrel, Bill and Pam. *Men Are Like Waffles, Women Are Like Spaghetti: Understanding and Delighting in Your Differences.* Harvest House, 2001.

Fernandez, Alvaro, and Elkhonon Goldberg with Pascale Michelon, *The SharpBrains Guide to Brain Fitness: How To Optimize Brain Health and Performance at Any Age.* 2nd ed. SharpBrains Incorporated, 2013.

Fuhrman, Joel. *Eat to Live: The Amazing Nutrient-Rich Program for Fast and Sustained Weight Loss.* Little, Brown and Company, 2003.

Genova, Lisa. *Still Alice.* Gallery Books, 2009.

Goff, Bob. *Love Does: Discover a Secretly Incredible Life in an Ordinary World.* Thomas Nelson, 2012.

Goleman, Daniel. *Emotional Intelligence: Why It Can Matter More than IQ.* Bantam Books, 1995.

    Focus: The Hidden Driver of Excellence. HarperCollins, 2013.

    Social Intelligence: The Revolutionary New Science of Human Relationships. Bantam, 2006.

Gray, John. *Men Are from Mars, Women Are from Venus: A Practical Guide for Improving Communication and Getting What You Want in Your Relationships.* HarperCollins, 1992.

Gungor, Mark. "Tale of Two Brains: Unlocking the Secrets to Life, Love and Marriage." DVD. Laugh Your Way America, 2007.

Haase, Albert. *Catching Fire, Becoming Flame: A Guide for Spiritual Transformation.* Paraclete Press, 2013.

    This Sacred Moment: Becoming Holy Right Where You Are. Intervarsity Press, 2010.

Hannaford, Carla. *Smart Moves: Why Earning Is Not All in Your Head.* Great Ocean, 1995.

Hanson, Rick. *Hardwiring Happiness: The Practical Science of Reshaping Your Brain— and Your Life.* Rider, 2013.

Heagle, John. *Justice Rising: The Emerging Biblical Vision.* Orbis Books, 2010.

    Life to the Full, Thomas More Press, 1976.

Hiss, Kimberly. "The Beautiful Life of Your Brain." *Reader's Digest* (September 2014): 76-85.

Horstman, Judith. *The Scientific American Day in the Life of Your Brain: A 24-Hour Long Journal of What's Happening in Your Brain as You Sleep, Dream, Wake Up, Eat, Work, Play, Fight, Love, Worry, Compete, Hope, Make Important Decisions, Age, and Change.* Jossey-Bass, 2009.

Hyman, Mark. *The UltraMind Solution: Fix Your Broken Brain by Healing Your Body First.* Scribner, 2007.

Jensen, Eric. *Music with the Brain in Mind.* Corwin, 2000.

Johnson, Sue, and Julie Carlson. *Grandloving: Making Memories with Your Grandchildren.* Heartstrings Press, 2000.

Johnson, Spencer. *The Precious Present.* Doubleday, 1984.

Katz, Lawrence C., and Manning Rubin. *Keep Your Brain Alive: 83 Neurobic Exercises to Help Prevent Memory Loss and Increase Mental Fitness.* Workman Publishing Company, 1999.

Klemko, Robert. "If You Give a Mouse a Concussion." *Sports Illustrated* (April 20, 2014): 40-43.

Lamott, Anne. *Help, Thanks, Wow: The Three Essential Prayers.* Riverhead Hardcover, 2012.

Leaf, Caroline. *Switch On Your Brain: The Key to Peak Happiness, Thinking, and Health.* Baker Books, 2013.

Lucado, Max. *In the Grip of Grace: You Can't Fall Beyond His Love.* Thomas Nelson, 1996.

Medina, John. *Brain Rules: 12 Principles for Surviving and Thriving at Work, Home, and School.* Pear Press, 2014.

Massachusetts General Hospital. *Mind, Mood & Memory.* (March 2011): 6; (June 2012): 4; (November, 2012): 6.

Nelson, Aaron P., and Susan Gilbert. *The Harvard Medical School Guide to Achieving Optimal Memory.* McGraw-Hill, 2005.

Pauley, Jane. *Your Life Calling: Reimagining the Rest of Your Life.* Simon & Schuster, 2014.

Ratey, John J., with Eric Hagerman. *Spark: The Revolutionary New Science of Exercise and the Brain.* Little, Brown and Company, 2008.
   A User's Guide to the Brain: Perception, Attention, and the Four Theaters of the Brain. Vintage, 2002.

Sapolsky, Robert M. *Why Zebras Don't Get Ulcers: The Acclaimed Guide to Stress, Stress-Related Diseases, and Coping.* Holt, 1998.

Sax, Leonard. *Why Gender Matters: What Parents and Teachers Need to Know About the Emerging Science of Sex Differences.* Doubleday, 2005.

Siegel, Daniel J. *The Developing Mind: How Relationships and the Brain Interact to Shape Who We Are.* 2nd ed. The Guilford Press, 2012.

Sood, Amit. *Train Your Brain, Engage Your Heart, Transform Your Life: A Two Step Program to Enhance Attention; Decrease Stress; Cultivate Peace, Joy and Resilience: and Practice Presence with Love.* Morning Dew, 2009.

Sweeney, Michael S. *Brain—The Complete Mind: How It Develops, How It Works, and How to Keep It Sharp.* National Geographic, 2009.

Sylwester, Robert. *How to Explain a Brain: An Educator's Handbook of Brain Terms and Cognitive Processes.* Corwin, 2004.

Taylor, Jill Bolte. *My Stroke of Insight: A Brain Scientist's Personal Journey.* Viking, 2006.

Voskamp, Ann. *One Thousand Gifts: A Dare to Live Fully Right Where You Are.* Zondervan, 2010.

Warren, Rick, Daniel Amen, and Mark Hyman. *The Daniel Plan: 40 Days to a Healthier Life.* Zondervan, 2013.

Weil, Andrew. *Spontaneous Happiness: A New Path to Emotional Well-Being.* Little, Brown and Company, 2013.

Zimmer, Carl. "Secrets of the Brain, New Technologies Are Shedding Light on Biology's Greatest Unsolved Mystery: How the Brain Really Works." *National Geographic* (February 2014): 28-57.

Websites and Online Resources

Alzheimer's Association website. www.alz.org

204 | MAX YOUR MIND

The American Institute of Stress website. http://www.stress.org/daily-life/
"50 Common Signs and Symptoms of Stress." http://www.stress.org/stress-effects/#sthash.5BYq9Fjt.dpuf
Brain Connection website. http://brainconnection.brainhq.com/
Edu-Kinesthetics, Inc. Brain Gym website. www.braingym.com
The Franklin Institute. "Nourish: Proteins." Human Brain website. http://learn.fi.edu/learn/brain/proteins.html
Kovacs, Jenny Stamos. "Beans: Protein-Rich Superfoods." WebMD. March 1, 2007. http://www.webmd.com/diet/features/beans-protein-rich-superfoods
National Sleep Foundation website. http://sleepfoundation.org
"Ask the Expert: Can Exercise Help with Excessive Sleepiness?" Dr. Barbara Phillips, expert. February 25, 2013. http://sleepfoundation.org/ask-the-expert/can-exercise-help-excessive-sleepiness
"Caffeine and Sleep." Reviewed by Dr. Greg Belenky. http://sleepfoundation.org/sleep-topics/caffeine-and-sleep
"Healthy Sleep Tips." http://sleepfoundation.org/sleep-tools-tips/healthy-sleep-tips/page/0%2C1/
"The Neuroscience of Finding Your Lost Keys." ScienceBlog website. March 21, 2013. http://scienceblog.com/61618/the-neuroscience-of-finding-your-lost-keys/#jVoGf5jeI1xGvoeO.99
Paddock, Catharine. "Sleep Helps 'Detox' Your Brain." The Center for Sleep Medicine website. http://www.chicagosleepstudy.com/sleep_helps_detox_your_brain.html
Voskamp, Ann. www.aholyexperience.com

ACKNOWLEDGMENTS

Writing a book is clearly a team project. This dream began with a hunger God gave me to make sense of our miraculous brains and help others improve their lives with the insights. The people and experiences he placed in my life have shaped and guided the project.

My gratitude flies out to many special people as I reflect on the years of this book's development. This work stands on the shoulders of countless researchers, spiritual leaders, and professional colleagues whose work provides the foundation for all of my own. My first psychology professor, Johanna Warloski at University of Wisconsin-Eau Claire, gave me a glimpse of the answers I was seeking. Professors at University of Wisconsin-Stout's Guidance and Counseling Program further guided my search and experiences. Special thanks to all the authors cited in *Max Your Mind*. You continue to teach me as I study your works: Aaron Nelson, PhD; Judith Horstman; Dan Goleman; Richard Davidson, PhD; Nancy C. Andreasen, PhD; Dr. Caroline Leaf; Willy Wood; John Medina; Mark Hyman; Diane Gossen; Ann Voskamp; and LeeAnna Rasar.

Schools have been golden opportunities for me to learn how the brain works and to work with staff, students, and families to develop brain-friendly programming. I've appreciated working together with counseling colleagues, families, students, and staff in each setting: Bitburg American Dependent School in Germany; Osseo-Fairchild, Wisconsin; Longfellow Elementary and Putnam Heights of the Eau Claire Area School District; and Kunming International Academy. I learned a great deal within the mutually supportive atmosphere in each school setting. Updated versions of these programs continue to support healthy development and relationships.

Counseling colleagues, families, students, and staff in Bitburg American Dependent School in Germany; Osseo-Fairchild, Wisconsin; Eau Claire Area School District; and Kunming International Academy all contributed support, patience, mentorship, appreciation, and stepping stones to help me find the brain-coaching answers I was seeking.

The Wisconsin School Counselor Association was a gold mine of resources, contacts, and professional networking and support. I appreciate your service as a sounding board for these developing ideas. Kudos to my former practicum student, colleague, and friend, Kelly Curtis, who continues the proud WSCA tradition serving as their current president.

For fifteen years, our collaborative BRAIN Team professionals kept me in touch with ongoing neuroscience developments and gave me opportunities to share meaningful current research and best practices with the people who can benefit from applying the information to their lives. I thank them and the Wisconsin Council for Children and Families for training and mutual support.

Organizations who hosted my presentations gave me the incentive I needed to put all the research together into digestible, clear messages that became central elements of this book. My appreciation goes to each of them, including Health Ed Inc., Family Resource Center of Eau Claire, the Alberta, Canada, Special Education Association, and many others. Preparing for each group led me to new answers and still more questions, moving me along my journey. I thank you!

The writing professionals I've met at conferences have shown me the best ways to download the information I've gathered over so many years. At Write to Publish, I met author and mentor Virelle Kidder, who led me gently and steadily through the Christian Writers Guild Apprentice Course. Countless times I wanted to give up, but she always pulled me back from the brink. Bless you, my friend! You have shaped and grown my writing beyond what I could have imagined.

Thanks to Sandra Bishop, who reviewed an early draft of this project and made very helpful recommendations. You pointed me in the right direction, and I thank you. Kathy Carlton Willis and the Western Wisconsin Christian Writers Guild offered significant training and guidance as I began publishing in magazines as a foundation for creating this book.

Terry Whalin recognized and encouraged this vision many years ago during conferences. Reconnecting with him this year restored my enthusiasm to carry the project forward to Morgan James Publishing. I appreciated meeting the Morgan James family at the Author 101 University conference in March, and their guidance through the many steps along the way. I'm so thankful to have met my enthusiastic and hopeful friend Vera during that conference. She continues to be my spiritual blessing as we share beliefs about personal purpose and success. When my husband and I began our recent European vacation, she gifted us with a personal walking and canal tour of Amsterdam. We continue our spiritual connection, although an ocean apart.

Sheri Baemmert's technological and artistic expertise and emergency rescues have enhanced the project's visual elements and preserved my sense of peace. How convenient to have both graphic artist and Pilate's trainer wrapped into one gifted woman! Her targeted Pilate's workouts ease my body's protests from all the computer hours. Robin's massages kept fibromyalgia from interrupting my writing. You have both kept this project afloat.

Spiritual guidance for this project began with Rev. Erling Carlsen in Cumberland, and continued with Fr. John Heagle's and Fr. George Szew's reflections and direction. My appreciation goes to Rev. Mark Schultz, Lynette Schultz, and my dear Peace Lutheran Small Group prayer partners who refresh my soul each week during our Bible Study.

Amanda Rooker and her SplitSeed editing staff kept my focus on the Source of the inspiration for Max Your Mind and kept my words meaningful and inviting for readers. With each editing conference, she reminds me that this is God's project. Its path, purpose, and mission begin and end with him—not me. What a comfort that is! I will be forever grateful to her for teaching and guiding me to my best writing. Serving as a conduit for his message through my words has many mornings left me breathless and so blessed!

Morgan James Publishing and their author-centric processes have been very helpful throughout the book's development. I appreciate the opportunity to dialogue about the book to provide the best experience for readers.

Such an ambitious project could not be completed without knowledgeable readers who raise questions and maintain clarity for other readers. Special thanks for sharing your expertise go to Blythe Rinaldi, Lee Anna Rasar, Rosie Turcotte, Eric Alfrey, Fr. John Heagle, Fr. Albert Haase, Julie Manas, Ann Kaiser, Megan Turner, Jodi Ritsch, and Ann Brand.

My gratitude to friends who allowed me to share their stories to bring these principles to life: Tom and Mary Jo, Sue, Diann and Tom, Barb and Randy, Eula, Mike, and Mary.

Without my supportive family this book wouldn't have been possible. My husband of forty-eight years has done everything in his power to support me in this project. Special gratitude to our daughters, Dawn, Jen, and Heidi, their husbands, and our nine grandchildren, whose enthusiasm for my writing encouraged me through the long process.

My late mother and father, Marie and Herb Sunquist, believed in me from the start and would be proud to know it's finally happening. My sister Pam reminds me of her prayers every time we talk, and I've leaned hard on them throughout this project and my life. Our late brother Doug inspired me with his dedication to his own dream, even though it was cut short at a young age.

Phone conversations with Mom's sister, Lois Seldon, have kept me laughing and seeing God in the details of each step of this process. You've been an amazing gift, especially since Mom's passing. Mom was always proud of my helping people, and her best friend, Shirley Miller, reminds me of her dedication to supporting me in that effort.

My cousin Sylvia and I have been soul mates, sharing our birthday celebrations since we were small. Thanks for many reminders of your support for this vision over the years! Sustaining, long-term, unconditional friends Jean, Mickey, Sue, Kathy, Nancy, and Colleen have kept my spirit balanced even when circumstances threatened to throw me overboard.

The Marshfield Clinic Cancer Center staff has shown us the depth of God's love through Bob's and my cancer journeys. We agree with Diann and Tom who call you our angels. Our eternal gratitude goes to each person whose prayers carried us through our cancer journey. You know who you are, and we have already thanked you personally for your support.

Our oncologist recommended, "Plan another trip; they clearly agree with you!" We followed his orders and have come to know delightful friends on our travels, including Sally and Barry, Tom and Mary Jo, Marie and Gerry, Ursula and Fred, Curt and Mary, Bruce and Brenda, and Lori and Kevin. Thanks, each of you, for the laughter, your friendship, and your interest in this project!

The laughter and prayers of good friends help me stay physically and mentally healthy despite cancer and many other struggles. Good friends help keep my perspective without taking myself too seriously. Water Babes' laughter during pool workouts, coffee, and birthday celebrations keep me from taking myself too seriously. Peace Small Group friends and their prayers have kept my spirit moving toward hope.

I can't find the right words to thank long-term friends Nancy, Jean, Kathy, Susie, Mickey, Sue, Donna, Barb, Anne, and Colleen for caring enough to pull me back to the project when it felt hopeless. Friends and creative professional colleagues at The Center—Ann, Jodi, Lisa, Aveen, Judy, Scott, and Anita—have supported this project throughout its life. New friends within the Polkadot Powerhouse Dots keep encouraging my business growth and creativity.

Individual coaching clients inspire me with their courage and persistence in facing and overcoming challenges and creating their new lives. Sharing your journey has been an honor, inspiration, and joy for me.

Thanks to the group of former students and their parents who wrote stories for this book's initial plan. God may still have a purpose for them in future works.

Special thanks to readers who want to know more about their brain — without you, this book wouldn't have a purpose. I am eternally grateful for you and your journey. May you find your answers and the life you are seeking.

ABOUT THE AUTHOR

Sandra Sunquist Stanton, NCC, LPC, BCC, of Eau Claire, Wisconsin, is an author, speaker, professional counselor, certified coach, parent, wife, and grandma to nine amazing kids. Her alphabet soup of credentials translates to: Nationally Certified Counselor, Licensed Professional Counselor, and Board Certified Coach. She has helped people of all ages make the most of their amazing brains through her business, Connections of the Heart, LLC, which can be found on www.SandraStantonAuthor.com and www.ourbrainbuddies.com, Facebook, Twitter, LinkedIn, Google+, YouTube, Goodreads, and Pinterest. Sandra was invited to set up a guidance program at Kunming International Academy in Yunnan, China, has published over 50 articles and book chapters, and has presented more than 100 workshops in the US and Canada since retiring from a school counseling career that spanned twenty-five years.